T0270515

THE
COMPLETE
GUIDE TO
ALLERGIES

THE
COMPLETE
GUIDE TO
ALLERGIES

Recognizing and Treating Today's Most Common and Unusual Allergens

Dr. Catherine Quéquet
Translated by Grace McQuillan

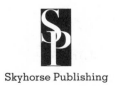

Skyhorse Publishing

Original French edition:
Les Nouvelles Allergies, Comment les reconnaître ? Comment les combattre ?
© 2022, Groupe Elidia Éditions du Rocher
28, rue Comte Félix-Gastaldi—BP 521—98 015 Monaco
www.editionsdurocher.fr

English translation copyright © 2024 Skyhorse Publishing
First Skyhorse Publishing edition, 2024

Skyhorse Publishing books may be purchased in bulk at special discounts for sales promotion, corporate gifts, fund-raising, or educational purposes. Special editions can also be created to specifications. For details, contact the Special Sales Department, Skyhorse Publishing, 307 West 36th Street, 11th Floor, New York, NY 10018 or info@skyhorsepublishing.com.

Skyhorse® and Skyhorse Publishing® are registered trademarks of Skyhorse Publishing, Inc.®, a Delaware corporation.

Visit our website at www.skyhorsepublishing.com.

10 9 8 7 6 5 4 3 2 1

Library of Congress Cataloging-in-Publication Data is available on file.

Cover design by David Ter-Avanesyan
Cover photo credit: Getty Images

Print ISBN: 978-1-5107-7396-7
Ebook ISBN: 978-1-5107-7397-4

Printed in the United States of America

Contents

Introduction

"I said 'bizarre,' did I? How bizarre!" Louis Jouvet's famous line from the French comedy *Bizarre, Bizarre* is exactly how most people react when they hear about certain allergies. Everyone has their own collection of stereotypes and knowledge about allergies, but these preconceptions are not always correct. In this book, we'll take an (often playful) look at all things allergies that you may never have believed possible. Studying allergies is an incredible adventure, and one that is becoming even more astonishing as the field continues to evolve. A quick glance through recent studies on the subject will give you ample proof that these strange allergies and triggers are growing in number. Were you aware, for instance, that sexual intercourse can cause an allergic reaction? Oh, and you think you know everything there is to know about dust mites? Well, did you have any idea that they are capable of migrating from one room to another? Medical journal articles are filled with these kinds of oddities: sperm, beer, caviar, cannabis, surfing, gold . . . you name it! Researchers are learning more and more about these emerging allergies and what triggers them, so why wouldn't I share their discoveries with you? I'd like to invite you to explore the lesser-known side of these allergies and their major players. The information in this book will prove essential to helping you better understand modern allergies and how to manage them.

PART ONE
EXPLORING NEW ALLERGIES

CHAPTER 1

What Is an Allergy?

An allergy is the body's inappropriate and exaggerated reaction to substances in its environment. Before you continue reading, it's important for me to mention that there are several kinds of allergies, not just one. The term "allergy" (*allos*: "other," *ergon*: "reaction") was first used by Austrian pediatrician Clemens von Pirquet in 1906. He defined it as "the state of an individual who, after sensitization to a substance (allergen), subsequently reacts to it in exaggerated fashion."

Immediate IgE-mediated respiratory and food allergies

If you listen to people talk about allergies, they very likely mention things like "rhinitis," "conjunctivitis," "asthma," "food allergies," and "anaphylactic shock." All of these are indications that the allergic individual, when triggered, experiences a series of immediate reactions termed "IgE-dependent" or "IgE-mediated." Some people are genetically predisposed to these hypersensitive reactions to their environment; they are said to be "atopic." This is why it is important to find out about any allergies in your family history.

In spite of this predisposition, an atopic individual does not develop an allergy by chance, but rather because he or she is able to produce specific immunoglobulin E (IgE) antibodies for proteins (allergens) found in dust mites, animals, certain foods, pollens, etc. The common misconception that an allergy can appear overnight is utterly inaccurate because there is always an initial period of "sensitization." During this preliminary phase, the body is exposed to an allergen and produces IgE antibodies for it without triggering any symptoms. This period can vary in length from a few months to several years. When the body is later reexposed to that same allergen, the IgE antibodies cause an allergic response along with an entire cortege of symptoms, which vary depending on the allergen. The first signs may be skin and tissue related (eczema, hives, angioedema), respiratory (allergic rhinitis, asthma), or, in the case of anaphylactic shock, symptoms are more generalized and affect multiple organ systems.

Atopic risk according to Kjellman (1977)
- 12% for a child if neither parent has allergies
- 20% if one parent has allergies
- 43% if both parents have allergies
- 72% if both parents have the same kind of allergy

IgE-mediated allergic reactions are generally described as "immediate" because the symptoms mentioned above are rapidly triggered in the minutes or hours following exposure to the allergen. This timeline is of tremendous importance during the process of diagnosing an allergy, particularly those related to food. I should note here that not all IgE-mediated food allergies cause immediate symptoms. There are two notable exceptions—alpha-gal syndrome (or mammalian meat allergy) and natto allergy—and we'll come back to them later.

The **diagnosis** of these kinds of allergies typically follows the same set of steps. It begins with a meticulous, almost inter-rogation-like interview with an allergist. This gives the doctor information that will guide future testing. People decide to consult an allergy specialist for many different reasons. Perhaps they're suffering from a permanent case of rhinitis, which is often linked to the presence of dust mites, pets, or mold in the home. Others may experience seasonal allergies every year when they come into repeated contact with various types of pollen. "Hay fever" triggered by grass seed pollen is the best-known exam-ple and causes coughing, wheezing, and other ear-nose-throat symptoms.

Skin allergies, by contrast, may manifest as patches of eczema spread over the entire body in children, or as cycles of eczema flare-ups followed by remission in adults. It is now established that atopic dermatitis (eczema) flare-ups are not caused by a food allergy. In fact, the reverse is true: fragile, irritated skin can allow the body to become sensitized and later allergic to certain foods.

The entourage of food allergy symptoms includes, among other things, local or generalized hives, sometimes accompanied by angioedema. The primary symptom of a severe allergy, however, is still the dreaded anaphylaxis. Since food allergens are not the only cause of anaphylaxis, it's important not to rule out certain medications (antibiotics, muscle relaxants) and insect stings (wasp, bee, hornet) during an allergy diagnosis.

In an emergency situation, the diagnosis of anaphylaxis is highly likely if at least one of these three criteria* is met:

1: Acute onset of an illness (minutes to several hours) with simultaneous involvement of the skin, mucosal tissue, or both (e.g., generalized hives, pruritus or flushing, swollen lips-tongue-uvula) with no known exposure to an allergen.
   a. Respiratory compromise (e.g., dyspnea, wheeze-bronchospasm, stridor, reduced peak expiratory flow (PEF), hypoxemia).
   b. Reduced blood pressure (systolic blood pressure <90 mmHg) or associated symptoms of end-organ dysfunction (e.g., hypotonia [collapse], syncope, incontinence).

World Allergy Organization Anaphylaxis Guidance 2020

To illustrate this, let's imagine the case of adult X or child Y. Over the course of a meal (or in the minutes or hours that follow it), X or Y finds themselves covered with itchy red bumps (hives, pruritus) and notices that their lips are swollen

---

* Known as the Sampson Criteria.

(angioedema). At first, he or she does not understand what is happening. If these symptoms are accompanied by shortness of breath (dyspnea), wheezing (bronchospasm), or a high-pitched whine coming from the back of the throat (stridor), anaphylaxis is extremely likely. Later, when their lung function is being measured in the emergency room, the medical team may also observe a drop in oxygen levels (hypoxemia) and a decreased flow of air when the patient exhales. It's important to remember that an asthma attack with bronchospasm triggered by a food allergy is actually a sign of anaphylaxis and should be treated with an injection of epinephrine, not with the bronchodilators used during a classic asthma attack brought on by airborne allergens.* The final symptom mentioned above—X's or Y's low blood pressure—will cause dizziness and could lead to a coma.

2: Two or more symptoms after exposure to a probable allergen:
   a. Skin/mucosal tissue involvement (hives, pruritus or flushing, swollen lips-tongue-uvula).
   b. Respiratory compromise (e.g., dyspnea, wheeze-bronchospasm, stridor, reduced peak expiratory flow (PEF), hypoxemia).
   c. Reduced blood pressure (systolic blood pressure <90 mmHg) or onset of hypotension (decrease in systolic blood pressure greater than 30 percent from that person's baseline).
   d. Persistent gastrointestinal symptoms (abdominal pain, vomiting).

---

* Dust mites, animals, pollen, mold.

World Allergy Organization Anaphylaxis Guidance 2020

In the second situation presented above, Mr. or Mrs. X or child Y thinks they may have eaten something they are allergic to during the meal. This could happen if, for example, an allergic individual consumes packaged foods without checking the label beforehand, but it can also happen as a result of indirect contamination or contact with allergens present on another person's body. This will be discussed in more detail later on.

> 3: Systolic blood pressure below 90 mmHg or a decrease greater than 30 percent from an adult's baseline blood pressure after exposure to a known allergen. In children, systolic blood pressure may drop below 70 mmHg.

World Allergy Organization Anaphylaxis Guidance 2020

In this third scenario, Mr. or Mrs. X or child Y knows for certain that they have ingested a food they are allergic to.

There are certain early warning signs that will alert an allergic individual that their reaction is getting worse and prompt them to self-inject with epinephrine before calling 911. They may feel tingling in their hands or feet or notice a metallic taste in their mouth, their voice may sound hoarse, and they may experience nausea, vomiting, or a headache.

On the other hand, if these symptoms appear in a person who has never had these kinds of reactions beforehand, the first thing to do is lay them down in the recovery position and call

911. Most importantly, do not drive the person to the emergency room—wait for an ambulance and medical advice.

Important Emergency Information

Many of the cases described in this book involve anaphylaxis. Emergency treatment of this kind of reaction requires an intramuscular injection of epinephrine on the outer thigh and hospitalization for at least seven hours of monitoring. This is why people with known or diagnosed allergies should *always* carry an epinephrine auto-injector, commonly known as an EpiPen.

Allergy testing should never be undertaken during a pregnancy (out of precaution), an acute allergic reaction (to avoid making it worse), or while a person is taking antihistamines (they reduce the skin's reactivity and could distort test results). Testing should also be at least four to six weeks after anaphylaxis (a shorter length of time risks a repeat episode). Skin prick tests, as they are known, are used only for immediate allergies. An allergy is diagnosed when there is an observed connection between the allergic events in the patient's medical history and prick positivity. These tests are reliable, reproducible, and painless. The skin is pricked with a small needle and a drop of allergen is introduced without causing any bleeding. Fifteen to twenty minutes later, the test is read. A test is considered positive if a raised bump and redness have appeared where the allergen extract was deposited. Contrary to popular belief, skin prick tests for food allergies can be performed on babies as young as one month old. They can be used to test for respiratory allergies a little later when a child is around two and a half or three years old. The choice of which allergens to test will depend on the information provided during the initial patient interview.

Intradermal allergy tests (IDT) are small injections below the surface of the skin of progressively larger allergen concentrations (this is the same technique used for injecting tuberculin during a tuberculosis skin test). IDTs are normally only used for diagnosing drug or insect venom allergies and should be performed by a specialist in a medical facility.

When it comes to diagnosing a food allergy, tests called oral food challenges (OFC) can be extremely helpful. These tests have several objectives:

- Definitive diagnosis: identifying exactly which food allergen is causing problems for a patient is especially important when that patient has multiple allergies, which is a more and more frequent problem.
- Determine a patient's reactivity threshold: oral food challenges will demonstrate whether an allergic individual can safely eat products containing traces of the allergen without or if they should avoid them completely. This threshold also helps allergists map out future oral immunotherapy treatment.
- Evaluate how well a patient is responding to treatment: after an initial oral food challenge, treatments like oral immunotherapy can begin. Oral immunotherapy (OIT)

aims to train the body to accept the food allergen by reintroducing it into the patient's diet little by little. Ideally, the patient will eventually be able to consume normal amounts of the food allergen on a regular basis. Oral food challenges may be given during the course of OIT to determine if treatment has been successful.

Oral immunotherapy is a food desensitization treatment recommended for children and young adults. An allergist may suggest starting OIT after an oral food challenge. Treatment follows a strict protocol and involves daily ingestion of small, slowly increasing amounts of the once forbidden food over the course of several months. Patients with a history of anaphylaxis are not eligible for oral immunotherapy and this treatment should never be attempted at home without medical advice. Regular consultations with an allergist for OFC monitoring will determine if the dose or length of time between doses should be adjusted. For the moment, oral immunotherapy is not offered for all food allergens and the majority of research has focused on its effectiveness for peanut and dairy allergies.

Drugs known as biologics that target IgE antibodies offer another useful allergy treatment, particularly for patients with multiple allergies and what we call cross-reactivities.*

People used to say that a person was allergic "to cats," "to milk," or "to eggs." Over the years, diagnostic techniques and immunology research have improved, and we can now identify

---

* This happens when two different substances have a similar molecular structure.

with far greater precision which allergens are responsible for a reaction. Some allergens, for instance, are sensitive to the way a certain food is cooked and digested. Knowing how a food allergen behaves when it is consumed raw or cooked is the kind of valuable information an allergist uses to set up an elimination diet.

To illustrate how important this highly specific knowledge of allergens can be, let's take the case of people who are allergic to apples but can eat them cooked in a pie, applesauce, or jam with no problem at all. These people react to proteins in the PR-10 family (plant defense proteins) that are destroyed when the fruit is cooked. For them, eating those same apples raw would trigger itchy mouth or swelling of the lips. People with this allergy also often react to birch tree pollen in a cross-reactivity known as pollen-food allergy syndrome.

Researchers have also been able to pinpoint that there are two major allergens in egg whites that react to heat in completely different ways. Ovalbumin is destroyed during cooking, whereas ovomucoid is heat resistant. For people allergic to egg whites, this is an important distinction to be aware of!

As new allergens are discovered, each one is assigned a name in accordance with IUIS* nomenclature rules. This name consists of the first three letters of the genus, the first letter of the species, and a number indicating the order of discovery.

Here are a few examples:

---

* International Union of Immunological Societies.

- Birch tree pollen: Betv1 = Betula verrucosa 1 for the first allergen discovered.
- Peanuts: Arah1 = Arachis hypogea 1. This is followed by Arah2, Arah3, Arah8, and Arah9.
- Cats: Feld1 = Felis domesticus 1.

Allergens are also classified as either major or minor allergens. A major allergen, as you might imagine, is a protein that triggers allergic reactions in more than 50 percent of allergic individuals. A minor allergen, then, is one that concerns less than 50 percent of this population.

For example: the cat allergen Feld1 is a major allergen since more than 90 percent of people allergic to cats react to it. Feld2, on the other hand, is a minor allergen because it produces a reaction in less than 50 percent of people allergic to cats.

Non–IgE–mediated allergic contact dermatitis

In the following list, you'll find what makes contact allergies different from the allergies discussed earlier in this chapter:

- There is a longer delay (at least forty-eight hours) between exposure to the allergen (cosmetics, industrial materials, etc.) and the first appearance of symptoms.
- The reaction follows an entirely different immunological mechanism.

- Specific IgE antibodies do not play a role in a contact dermatitis reaction and the individual experiencing symptoms is not necessarily atopic.
- Symptoms of contact dermatitis (a form of eczema) can range from dry, red patches that get worse with continued allergen contact to more severe cases with cysts and blisters, oozing, and bacterial infection.
- It is also important to remember that there is a difference between skin that is irritated by exposure to something (an ingredient in a cosmetic product, for example) and skin that is having an allergic reaction to a particular substance.

ALLERGY OR IRRITATION?

	Irritation	Allergy
Tightness	Yes	No
Tingling	Yes	No
Burning	Yes	No
Itching	No	Yes + +
Redness	Yes	Yes
Swelling	Yes	Yes
Dry, flaky skin (desquamation)	Yes	Yes
Small blisters	No	Yes
Cracked skin	Yes	No

Allergy testing always begins with these very important questions: where, when, how, and with what?

So, with that in mind, remember this piece of advice: if you ever have these kinds of reactions to cosmetics or any other product, don't just throw them in the trash. Instead, bring them to your doctor's appointment, with the original packaging if possible.

Patch testing can help find out what is causing a case of contact dermatitis. First, your doctor will place small amounts of allergens on your skin and cover them with a patch. At a second appointment forty-eight to seventy-two hours later, he or she will look at which allergens produced a reaction. Patch tests can also be done with samples of personal products that the patient brings in (though this does depend on the item's composition and pH). If traditional patch testing is not yielding clear results about what product is causing the skin issues, your doctor may propose repeated open application testing (ROAT).

Non-IgE-mediated food allergies

We saw earlier that most food allergies are IgE-mediated. There are, however, other forms of food allergies that affect the gastrointestinal tract and follow more complex non-IgE-mediated mechanisms. FPIES* is one example. Though first described in 1967, it was not until much later that scientists recognized it as an immune system issue. Another condition, eosinophilic esophagitis (EoE), first appeared in publications in 1981, but its exact mechanism is still not fully understood. What we do know is that milk proteins appear to have a unique ability to trigger non-IgE-mediated allergic reactions involving the skin (eczema) and/or digestive system, causing bloating, reflux, and chronic

---

* Food protein-induced enterocolitis syndrome.

diarrhea that, if left untreated, causes severe weight loss.* We will discuss this in greater detail later.

Hives

Regardless of what causes them (an allergy or any number of other things), hives are always characterized by the temporary or chronic appearance of a red rash. This rash may also itch and resemble a stinging nettle rash with raised bumps. Hives are sometimes accompanied by swelling of the lips or eyelids.

The number of people with food allergies is constantly on the rise, and the triggers for these issues are becoming increasingly nuanced. Therefore, you should keep in mind what we discuss throughout the rest of this book about these new allergies and their unusual causes—this information could be helpful for you or someone you know in the future.

---

*   Failure to thrive.

CHAPTER 2

The Gut Microbiome, Dysbiosis, and Allergies

Our airways, skin, and gastrointestinal tract are populated by a variety of microorganisms that live in harmony with our bodies most of the time. But when these microorganisms are disrupted and thrown off balance, they rebel, and diseases like allergies and asthma rear their heads. Because of this, we have to take extra special care of these little creatures. In this chapter we will focus primarily on the gut microbiome (also referred to as "intestinal flora") because it plays such an important role in allergy development. Before we do that, though, let's go over a few things about gut health.

Bloating and gas that feels ready to escape if you move so much as an inch can make life unpleasant. You know the feeling: that sudden obligation to squeeze your cheeks together to keep anything from escaping during a work meeting, that little fart asking only to be released. Sometimes it's able to make its way out discreetly. But other times it is accompanied by a soft and subtle sound, a kind of "pfiuut" that only a trained ear can detect. And sometimes it's a sudden roar that makes your seat vibrate, unleashing hysterical laughter from everyone around you. And let's not even talk about that moment in the elevator when, without too much noise, a pestilential odor suddenly seeps out and all of the passengers look around at each other silently wondering who is responsible.

Perhaps, from time to time, you've also experienced what feels like your stomach being ground into pieces, gut-twisting pain that bends you in half and nails you to your bed. When this happens, no antispasmodic worthy of its name is able to relieve your symptoms.

And then there's the urgent need to run to the bathroom—how could I forget? The diarrhea that arrives unannounced, without an appointment, sneaking in to upset your plans for the day.

If that wasn't distressing enough, there's always the chance someone will ask you when your baby is due, when the truth is that last night's dinner wreaked havoc on your gut microbiome and now your belly resembles a hot air balloon!

All of us have had to deal with at least one of these gut-related issues, and when these things happen, we always look for something to blame. We want to know what's causing the problem. The first place to look when trying to get to the bottom of these burbling phenomena is your diet. Every hypothesis should be explored, and then the battle can begin.

Food intolerance and NCGS (non-celiac gluten sensitivity)

In my career as an allergist, I have met many people who are suffering and come to me because they don't know where else to turn. These patients just want answers, and many of them want to believe that a food allergy is causing their problems because they're at their wits' end. Before coming to my office, many of them have already consulted a gastroenterologist with endoscopies and colonoscopies to prove it, but everything has come back normal. When this is the case, I know that with these patients I am not dealing with celiac disease or IBD*, both of which belong to the domain of gastroenterology.

> Celiac disease and gluten intolerance have nothing to do with wheat allergy. Celiac is an autoimmune disease where the ingestion of gluten, a protein found in wheat, rye, barley, spelt, and Kamut, prompts the body to attack the villi of the small intestine. As a result of this damage, micronutrients are malabsorbed and symptoms like diarrhea, intense fatigue, bloating, and anemia may be observed. Diagnosis usually requires an intestinal biopsy and blood tests to measure levels of tissue transglutaminase IgA antibodies.

In adult patients, except for those suffering from irritable bowel syndrome (IBS), the problem is often due to an intolerance. My role is to explore the allergy side of things to make sure every other possibility has been ruled out.

If the allergy tests are negative, I then have to explain to the patient that there are a number of nonallergic pathologies that

---

* Inflammatory bowel diseases, like ulcerative colitis and Crohn's disease.

could be causing their symptoms. These include lactose intolerance, non-celiac gluten sensitivity, and FODMAP intolerance (fermentable oligo-, di-, monosaccharides, and polyols).

Lactose intolerance

Normally, the lactase enzyme allows the body to split milk sugar (lactose) into glucose and galactose, two monosaccharides that are easier for the digestive tract to absorb. A deficit of this enzyme can cause problems for some people because lactose becomes extremely difficult for them to digest. This can cause bloating, gas, and diarrhea after the ingestion of dairy products or processed foods containing milk. We now know that this phenomenon affects people of different ethnic backgrounds in different ways.

> **Lactose Intolerance by Population Group**
> Central Europe: 2%–20%
> Mediterranean countries: 40%
> African continent: 65%–75%
> Asia: 90%

While lactose intolerance is not harmful in the majority of cases, its effects can be exacerbated if accompanied by other digestive disorders like gastroenteritis, colitis, celiac, or Crohn's. Symptoms may also develop after a round of antibiotics or chemotherapy. Alactasia, sometimes referred to as "congenital lactose intolerance," is a rare genetic disorder characterized by an almost complete absence of lactase activity from birth.

Non-celiac gluten sensitivity (NCGS)

The mechanism of non-celiac gluten sensitivity bears no resemblance to the mechanisms of wheat allergy or gluten intolerance (celiac disease). In fact, this condition is only diagnosed after these two other possibilities have been ruled out. NCGS causes symptoms like diarrhea, bloating, nausea, fatigue, and problems concentrating after gluten consumption. Everyone has his or her own gluten tolerance threshold, and in patients with NCGS, symptoms are triggered when this threshold is exceeded.

FODMAPs

This acronym stands for fermentable oligo-, di-, monosaccharides and polyols. The FODMAPs are short-chain carbohydrates found naturally in foods. In people sensitive to these carbohydrates, the FODMAPs are poorly or only partially digested by the small intestine. For these individuals, consuming FODMAPs can cause stomach discomfort, bloating, and altered bowel habits.

Non-IgE-mediated food allergies

In certain situations, gastroenterologists and allergists have to work together to diagnose non-IgE-mediated food allergies like eosinophilic esophagitis (EoE), eosinophilic gastroenteritis

(EGE), and FPIES (food protein-induced enterocolitis syndrome), many of which are misdiagnosed as other issues.

Eosinophilic Esophagitis (EoE)

This disorder is characterized by chronic inflammation of the esophagus and is diagnosed via endoscopy. The gastroenterologist performing the endoscopy will usually take a biopsy of the esophagus to verify an increased presence of eosinophils.[*] In young children, warning signs are bouts of vomiting, gastroesophageal reflux, and sometimes difficulty swallowing food.[**] Several foods may be responsible for this allergic response, both when eaten alone or with other foods. The six most frequent culprits are milk, wheat, legumes, eggs, fish, and seafood/shellfish. In these instances, collaboration between the gastroenterologist and the allergist is key.

Food protein-induced enterocolitis syndrome (FPIES)

Unfortunately, this food allergy is still poorly understood. In acute FPIES, patients present with projectile vomiting in the first three hours after ingesting the food allergen, which leads to severe dehydration, hypothermia, and a drop in blood pressure that requires emergency hospitalization. In its chronic form, the allergic reaction is characterized by intermittent vomiting, bloody diarrhea, and slight weight gain. While it is more common in children, it can develop in adults, as well.

---

*   Over 15 eosinophils per analyzed field.
** Dysphagia.

Non-IgE-mediated cow's milk protein allergy (CMPA)

Behind this diagnosis lies a hidden battle that many mothers are fighting every day. This allergy is often overlooked because health care professionals tend to focus on the immediate form of milk allergy rather than Non-Ige-mediated CMPA. Non-IgE-mediated CMPA causes skin issues (atopic eczema) as well as digestive symptoms, meaning parents need to pay close attention to both in very young children. Children with delayed allergic reactions to cow's milk protein may exhibit gastroesophageal reflux, bloating, and diarrhea that can lead to stunted growth if left unaddressed. Needless to say, this form of CMPA is often misdiagnosed and is a source of extreme anxiety for parents of children suffering from this food issue.[*]

The ABCs of digestion

I thought it might be a good idea to go back and take a look at human anatomy to explain the link between allergies and the digestive system. I could just draw you a picture of the digestive system with the small intestine (duodenum, jejunum, ileum), the large intestine (colon), etc. But I'm a little more interested in the microscopic side of things, getting up close and personal with our intestinal lining and food's marvelous voyage through our bodies: one day you're chewing it in your mouth, and just a few days later it's fecal matter—that's quite a journey!

---

[*] See page 83–84 in Chapter 3 for more information.

Let's be clear about this: I am in no way trying to pass myself off as a gastroenterologist. I'm simply going over the basics of digestion.

Eating is an undeniably essential part of our life. Our body needs calories, proteins, carbohydrates, and micronutrients to function correctly.

Biting, chewing, swallowing, and gulping down all kinds of foods is something we're used to doing. Every day, we make an appointment with our digestive tract. But when the machine starts to run haywire, nourishing our bodies becomes a daily struggle and sometimes leaves us having to loosen our belt buckle more often than we'd like.

Digestion is supposed to transform food so our bodies can absorb nutrients. What is the "alimentary bolus," you ask? Let's imagine it like a train leaving its point of origin, the mouth, and heading to its final destination, the anus. The passengers' names are simple sugars (lactose, fructose, saccharose, glucose), complex sugars (dietary fiber), proteins, lipids, minerals, vitamins, etc.

The train follows the tracks down the esophagus and into the stomach after the initial step of mastication (chewing). It continues moving forward thanks to small muscle contractions known as peristalsis. The stomach's stationmaster announces that some of the passengers will have to be tossed around and given a shower with hydrochloric acid to clean them off and make them easier to digest. They also have to pass muster with an array of enzymes. Then, after chugging through the pyloric sphincter, a kind of exit door at the bottom of the stomach, the locomotive enters the small intestine. This is where many "travelers" like amino acids and fatty acids get off the train to be absorbed by the microvilli on the intestinal lining. These villi are shaped like tiny roller coasters and offer over 250 square yards of surface area for nutrient absorption! The small intestine is also where lactose (milk sugar) is broken down into two more digestible molecules thanks to the lactase enzyme. If this enzyme's work is not up to par, the body will experience symptoms of lactose intolerance. Attacked by other enzymes, lipids transform into fatty acids. Proteins split into amino acids. All of these little travelers are metamorphosing into smaller molecules so the three portions of the small intestine can more readily absorb them. And they have plenty of time to do it, too: the small intestine is 19.5 to 22.5 feet long! Next, the food train heads toward the large intestine. The remaining passengers—water, fiber, and products not broken down in previous steps—will now be faced with the abundance of the gut microbiome, a veritable carpet of billions of microorganisms. This is where fecal matter formation happens and, if the circumstances are right, flammable gases will be produced along the way.

Our body is certainly one heck of a war machine, but when something goes awry, it leaves the owners of these machines in quite a bind. . . .

A few numbers
Small intestine: 19.5 to 22.5 feet
Large intestine (colon): 5 feet
The gut microbiome weighs 4.5 pounds
One gram of stool contains 100 billion bacteria

Millions of them

More and more researchers are focusing on the makeup of
the gut microbiome and its important role in allergy sensitivity. Epidemiological studies have shown that exposure to certain environmental elements can have a significant impact on
the microbiome's composition, and this in turn causes dysbiosis, which we can think of as a reshuffling or disorganization of
these otherwise friendly microorganisms.

Studies in mice have confirmed that the health of our gut
microbiome can determine our sensitivity or resistance to food
allergies. The researchers conducting these studies also identified a specific group of regulatory T-lymphocytes called FOXP3
(forkhead box P3) that plays a major role in immune tolerance.
This discovery paves the way for researching new, targeted
allergy treatments in the future. Why? Because these regulatory T-cells can modulate the balance between Th1 cells, which
fight bacterial infections, and Th2 cells, which respond to para-
site attacks. Higher levels of specialized Th2 and an imbalance
between these T-lymphocyte subgroups have been observed in
immediate IgE-mediated allergic responses to respiratory and
food allergens.

T-lymphocytes are white blood cells that play an important role
in the immune system's response to a variety of attacks. They are
produced in the bone marrow and mature in an organ called the
thymus located behind the sternum.

In the field of allergy medicine today, we are seeing the number of people with respiratory allergies starting to stagnate. Food allergy frequency, on the other hand, has exploded in recent years. There are many external factors that have something to do with this, as demonstrated by the effects of environment, diet, and the overuse of antibiotics on the health of the gut microbiome. The microbiome's equilibrium can also shift in response to products used in livestock breeding, or if our diet is too low in fiber. These microorganisms play a critical role in many of the body's processes and particularly in immune system function; they are involved in the synthesis of vitamins and immune-boosting short-chain fatty acids, dietary fiber digestion, and even the gut-brain axis.

These tiny inhabitants of the digestive tract first colonize our intestine when we are born and the microbiome reaches equilibrium at around age three. It includes fungi, bacteria, and viruses known as "phages," all of which prefer to grow in places devoid of oxygen. This constraint has led researchers in the last twenty years to develop new anaerobic culture methods (meaning without oxygen) as well as metabolite and genome analysis techniques that makes each microorganism easier to identify.

So how does this micropopulation get its start in life? It has the potential to do our body a great deal of good, but as we have seen, there are nefarious external factors that can get in the way and cause dysbiosis. As a reminder, dysbiosis is a state of imbalance characterized by a change in the health and abundance of the microbiome community. This is what increases a person's risk for developing allergies and asthma.

> The First 1,000 Days theory contends that everything that touches the fetus from conception until the age of two can have an impact on diseases that develop in the child's body later.

Initially, the newborn's digestive tract is sterile. Once a baby sticks its little nose out into the world, everything begins, and the gut's colonization by environmental bacteria is off to a running start.

Microbiome composition depends on many factors:

- Unlike a cesarean section, which takes place in a sterile operating room, vaginal birth offers the newborn plenty of microorganisms from the mother's genital area, from contact with the midwife or doctor delivering the baby, and their surroundings.
- Newborn feeding methods will also affect the extent to which the microbiome is stimulated and enriched. Exclusive breastfeeding provides a supply of microbes and other nutrients that prove significant when compared to bottle feeding with formula manufactured under (more or less) sterile conditions.

The choice of whether or not to breastfeed exclusively is a completely personal decision for every mother and the role it plays in preventing the development of future allergies is still up for debate, but breastfeeding does appear to be beneficial for the development of the baby's gut microbiome. If mothers decide to breastfeed their children, they should nevertheless be aware of one thing: breast-milk, on its own, does not contain beta-lactoglobulin proteins like those present in cow's milk. When a mother consumes dairy products, though, this food allergen is passed to her child via her breastmilk. As a result of this phenomenon, breastmilk can trigger cow's milk protein allergies in certain babies. This information is not meant to minimize the benefits of breastfeeding. On the contrary, understanding this possibility can point parents and doctors toward a cow's milk allergy diagnosis if an exclusively breastfed baby is experiencing digestive or skin issues.

The World Health Organization (WHO) recommends breastfeeding for at least six months. In atopic newborns, however, it's important to keep in mind that the early introduction of solid foods should take place during an oral tolerance window between the fourth and sixth month.

One thing is certain: breastfeeding, in concert with other environmental factors, has undeniable benefits for the diversity of the baby's gut microbiome.

Food tolerance develops best when a dense and diverse gut microbiome is already in place. Acquisition of this tolerance depends on early exposure to food allergens, ideally between the fourth and sixth month of life. Unfortunately, this perfect equilibrium can easily be thrown off balance. When a baby's diet prioritizes only certain kinds of foods and does not contain enough fiber, dysbiosis sets in and the diversity of the microbiome is altered. The development of food allergies is a sign of this physiological breakdown. Excessive and recurrent use of antibiotics, a diet low in fiber with overconsumption of omega-6 polyunsaturated fatty acids and alcohol (accompanied by triglyceride synthesis), and cesarean births are all part of the reason the gut microbiomes of people living in industrialized nations are in such poor condition. If we examine the microbiomes of atopic children more closely, the concentrations of bifidobacteria and lactobacilli* are astonishingly low. It is in precisely this context that allergy symptoms have a tendency to develop.

A recent study conducted in the United States showed that even though identical twins with allergies have identical genetic capital, they can nevertheless develop different food allergies depending on changes in the composition of their individual gut microbiomes.** Interestingly, healthy twins' gut microbiomes contain higher levels of clostridia bacteria (which protect against food allergies), *Phascolarctobacterium faecium*, and *Ruminococcus bromii*. This is only the beginning of the research that is needed in this area.

Food allergy is one of many diseases linked to changes in the gut microbiome. Others include obesity, diabetes, asthma, and autism. It is a field that continues to astound researchers and, in many ways, still remains a mystery.

---

* See definition on page 31.
** *Journal of Clinical Investigation.*

We now know that when the immune system is not stimulated early in life through contact with animals and microorganisms in the environment, this can lead to fluctuations in and depletion of the skin, respiratory, and gut microbiomes.

Luckily, there is some good news: the gut microbiome is a student that never stops trying. Even when it encounters disruptions and attacks from the outside, it can rebuild and be back to normal in a matter of weeks.

> The Human Microbiome Project (HMP) was a worldwide study launched with the aim of compiling the characteristics of the microorganisms that make up all of the body's microbiomes (oral, skin, vaginal, placental, gut).

Pre- and probiotics

Probiotics, as defined by the WHO, are "live microorganisms which when administered in adequate amounts confer a health benefit on the host." For the most part, these include lactobacilli and bifidobacteria, as well as yeasts like saccharomyces. Probiotics are used to treat or prevent diarrhea and IBD. In the past, they have also been recommended during pregnancy and breastfeeding, but there is no tangible evidence of their effectiveness in this area. The studies that have been published are hard to compare because the strains analyzed by each team of researchers are not the same and the clinical trials were not conducted in the same manner. Future publications will be better able to confirm whether or not probiotics are useful in allergy management.

Prebiotics, in the form of indigestible carbohydrates, provide the calories necessary for probiotic lactic acid bacteria to grow. The two work together in symbiosis. For the moment there are no recommendations for using these products on a regular basis, but certain possibilities are being studied.

CHAPTER 3

Unusual Allergies

As doctors, we must constantly keep learning about whatever new things are happening in our field. Reading scientific journals is part of this work. Whenever I flip through them—and there are many—my gaze tends to linger on certain clinical cases, ones that pique my curiosity, perplex me, and contain stories that are truly out of the ordinary. I thought it would be a wonderful idea to share them with you. This is my way, however small, of paying homage to all of the researchers and scientists who relentlessly publish their work to keep us informed. These real-life examples will also help you understand cross-reactivities and how an allergy is triggered in the first place (the phase of sensitization followed by the reaction phase). For people with allergies, they will be a source of additional information about substances and situations they may not usually view as risky, and if they observe new and unexplained allergy symptoms, the stories in this book will hopefully prompt them to make an appointment with their allergist. Some of you may not know you have an allergy. Perhaps you will recognize your symptoms in the cases presented here and decide to see an allergist to ask questions. There will be rhyming poems throughout this chapter to help you remember the most important information.

Inviting bees to your table is a bad idea

Before I tell this story, remember that the drone is the queen bee's "husband." It does not have a stinger and dies a few minutes after mating with the queen during their nuptial flight. Can you imagine if this happened in humans? It would mean the extinction of our species! The drone should also not be confused with the bumblebee, which plays an essential role as a pollinator.

I'll begin by saying this: Sometimes in life, people get strange ideas. While most of them are harmless, some can cause chaos.

Let's try not to panic!

The misadventures of a twenty-nine-year-old beekeeper are a perfect example. I have not embellished or added to the story that follows—believe me, it doesn't need it, and I've taken it straight from a medical journal. For an unknown reason, one day this young man decided to make himself a juice unlike any other. He takes out his juicer, gets everything ready, and starts juicing drone larvae! Yes, you read that right. When he pours himself a little glass of the beverage he has just concocted, he has no idea he is flirting with death. And yet . . .

Immediately after taking a sip, his mouth and ears start itching. You might be thinking that that was the end of it. But one hour later, he starts feeling worse. His body becomes covered in hives, he feels nauseated, and soon he starts vomiting and coughing. His face is completely swollen from angioedema and his heart is racing. Anaphylaxis is officially kicking in. When he arrives at the emergency room, he is treated with antihistamines and steroids. In my opinion, of course, he probably should have been given epinephrine! Either way, he stays at the hospital for a few hours to be monitored.

This beekeeper knows he is asthmatic. He has never shown signs of a bee or wasp allergy even though he has been stung over twenty times in the last two years. He is in total disbelief about what has just happened to him, especially since consuming royal jelly, honey, and propolis has never been a problem for him before.

The doctors try to determine how sensitization may have occurred, and conclude that their patient must have either ingested larvae residue without realizing it while harvesting royal jelly or inhaled particles of dust containing drone larvae during his beekeeping work.

Eating little critters

Let's take a glance at a new diet trend called entomophagy. The practice of eating insects is already widespread in Asia and South America, and the Food and Agriculture Organization of the

United Nations (FAO) estimates that 2.5 billion humans around the world consume insects on a regular basis.

Human consumption of this new kind of edible protein is becoming more and more frequent in Europe. Insects may sound like a perfectly harmless source of protein, but the number of serious allergic reactions that have been reported seems to indicate otherwise.

There is a known cross-reactivity between dust mites, mollusks, and other shellfish caused by a protein called tropomyosin. This same protein is present in edible insects, so it is certainly worth wondering what impact this new diet trend will have in Europe on the health of people with these kinds of allergies. In France, this trend has already made a timid appearance in the form of chocolate ants—depending on the recipe, these sweets may also feature mealworms and crickets!

The insects best known for this allergenic protein are mealworm larvae (*Tenebrio molitor*). They are high in protein (58.4 percent) and are used in sweet and savory dishes. In Mexico, for example, they are added to tortilla recipes. For real aficionados, in some places they can also be eaten live and are still extremely wiggly. Different insects are consumed in different countries depending on each culture's eating habits, but what is interesting for our purposes in this book is that if we add up all of the caterpillars, bees, ants, grasshoppers, crickets, hornets, and locusts that have been consumed, we also find several reported cases of anaphylaxis. In China, severe reactions after the ingestion of roasted silkworm pupa have been reported, and even caused the death of a French tourist in 2008. In 2012, another man tried to beat the sad record for the most cockroaches and worms eaten in one sitting. This challenge proved fatal a few hours later.

While many countries, like the United States, do not have laws against the consumption of insects (though the country does caution that insects consumed should be those specifically bred for human consumption), other countries do, in fact, have laws in place to keep its residents from consuming any and all insects. For example, a bulletin released on February 18, 2016, by the French Directorate General for Food (DGAL) confirms that it is illegal in France to a) feed livestock dead insects without prior processing and b) feed processed insect proteins to food-producing animals. Two years earlier, the French Directorate General for Competition Policy, Consumer Affairs, and Fraud Control (DGCCRF) had issued this reminder: "In the absence of current authorization for these commodities, they cannot be sold for human consumption." But are these measures being followed today? It would seem not: certain "mixtures" can be found in market stalls all over southern France.

French legislation may state that humans shouldn't eat insects, but they can easily be purchased on websites selling "specialty ingredients." The French Agency for Food, Environmental and Occupational Health & Safety (ANSES) warned insect eaters in April 2015 about the lack of clinical trials studying the risks involved with this kind of diet (infection, exposure to harmful chemicals) and formally condemned it. In sharp contrast, just one year before this warning, Belgium and its Federal Agency for the Safety of the Food Chain legalized the consumption of ten insects: the house cricket, the African migratory locust, the superworm, the yellow mealworm, the buffalo worm, the greater wax moth, the American desert locust, the banded cricket, the lesser wax moth, and the silk moth.

Since 2018, twenty-seven European countries have allowed edible insects (whole or parts) to be placed on the market for human consumption. All sales, however, must be approved by the European Commission in accordance with Regulation (EU) 2015/2283 concerning novel foods and "any food that was not used for human consumption to a significant degree within the Union before 15 May 1997." In spite of this trend toward tolerance, France has not yet warmed to the idea and continues to vigilantly monitor breeding and distribution methods.

Here's the moral of this story
As you can plainly see:
If allergies are what you've got
And you're worried, panic not!
But when you choose to eat "exotic"
Think twice or three times on the topic.
If it keeps you safe, it's not neurotic!

The surfer and the Japanese delicacy

Like Brice de Nice (from the French comedy directed by James Huth) or Patrick Swayze's Bodhi in *Point Break*, Fred is blond, tan, and muscular. He could easily be a runway or magazine model. But there's only one thing that interests him—no matter what time of year it is—and that's finding the best place on every continent to surf. The wave that will send the greatest shiver down his spine; the biggest adrenaline rush. On his board, he feels free. The only problem with this picture is that some beaches are swarming with jellyfish. These nasty gelatinous creatures can leave you with a stinging souvenir, and Fred has already run into quite a few of them throughout his travels.

Fred has the soul of an adventurer and has traveled the whole world with a surfboard under his arm. He eventually lands in Japan and decides to settle down in the coastal city of Shimoda. It should be noted that he has an incontestable weakness for Japanese culture. He knows everything about the local cuisine and particularly enjoys eating white rice served with natto, a dish he's quite fond of despite its off-putting odor and appearance. To each his own.

When our story begins, Fred has been complaining for a few weeks about waking up with itching and hives at around two or three o'clock in the morning. Then, one fateful night, he wakes up very out of breath. He can't breathe. He panics. His face is swollen, and despite how physically fit as he is, he suddenly feels extremely weak. Fred is going into anaphylactic shock. He owes his life to the quick action of his girlfriend, who happens to be a nurse, and an injection of epinephrine in the emergency room.

Because Fred's reaction was so severe, his doctors performed a thorough allergy investigation to determine what substance was responsible and to prevent it from happening again. One of them observed that Fred had eaten natto before each allergic episode. So what was causing his body's reaction?

The true story of natto allergy

When Naoko Inomata and his team published the first observation of this kind of anaphylactic allergy to natto in Japan in 2004, it sounded stranger than fiction. Their article described the case of an athletic man in his thirties who developed a severe allergic reaction ten hours after eating a dish of fermented soybeans.

This first case triggered a series of intensive research projects on this extraordinary subject. In time, a link was established between surfing (surfers are often attacked by jellyfish) and natto ingestion. The shared allergenic element was identified as poly(γ-glutamic acid) (PGA).

Natto is part of traditional Japanese cuisine. Here is the recipe, as explained by Yves, a French woman who has lived in Japan for several years: "The soybeans need to be soaked in water for over eight hours until softened. Then they are then boiled, and any white foam that forms on the surface of the water is removed. Most people suggest tasting the beans to know when they are done. . . . Then the bacteria for the natto are added, and the mixture is placed somewhere warm so that fermentation can take place."

By the time the dish is finished, the soybeans will have been cooked for twelve to twenty-four hours. PGA synthesis only begins once fermentation by *Bacillus subtilis* has taken place.

So then what exactly happened to poor Fred? Jellyfish tentacles are barbed with venomous organelles called nematocysts that are filled with PGA. When a surfer is stung by one of these brainless creatures, he or she becomes sensitized to this allergen. Other cnidarians, such as the sea anemone, also contain PGA.

There is still something that doesn't make sense. This allergy seems to occur more in surfers than in people who enjoy other water sports. Why? Researchers believe it could be because of the number of jellyfish on the surface of the water. Unlike windsurfing or boating, surfing puts the person in frequent direct contact with the water and, therefore, with jellyfish.

This hypothesis will have to be confirmed by additional studies.

Note

In the case of natto allergy, you may notice that the twelve-hour delay between its consumption and the appearance of symptoms differs from the classic food allergy model. Usually, in an immediate IgE-mediated allergic reaction, symptoms will appear within a few minutes or hours after ingestion. The reason the body takes longer to react to natto must be because of how slowly the molecules take to break down in order to be absorbed by the gastrointestinal lining.

Oodles of noodles . . . and PGA

Wait! Don't skip this paragraph! You don't have to be a nat-
to-eating surfer to be exposed to PGA! Because it is soluble in
water, it is often used in industrial and medical products including radiology contrast materials, as well as an ingredient in skin
moisturizers and exfoliants. In the food industry, PGA acts as
an acidity regulator or may be contained in food packaging. If
you happen to be traveling through parts of Asia or Australia,
you risk encountering another potential hazard: jellyfish salads.

What if only a small amount of PGA slips into something
like commercial Chinese noodles or soups? Unfortunately, as
we are about to see, that can be just as dangerous. A thirty-
eight-year-old man went to the store and bought a packaged
soup that contains cold Chinese noodles mixed with boiled
mung bean sprouts, leeks, and mustard. Three hours after
eating it, the first symptoms of anaphylaxis appeared. This
person had already been avoiding natto and all products
containing it for around three years because he always felt sick
the night after eating it. It had taken him around two years
to make the connection between natto and the severe allergic
reactions he was having.

After his reaction, skin prick tests were performed for all of
the ingredients he had consumed and the results were positive
for natto, the Chinese noodle soup, and PGA.

This information means that another diagnosis—MSG symptom complex, or "Chinese restaurant syndrome"—can be ruled
out. MSG symptom complex is connected to the consumption

of dishes containing monosodium glutamate (MSG), but our patient had no trouble eating this kind of food. After a thorough investigation, his doctors confirmed that the anaphylaxis was caused by PGA contained in the Chinese noodle soup. The noodle manufacturer was contacted and confirmed the presence of PGA in the dish. The patient was forced to stop all consumption of and contact with products containing this allergen. This means avoiding certain medications, breads, cookies, soups, sport drinks, and all soaps or creams that contain PGA.

There does not appear to be any direct correlation between natto allergy and allergies to soy or soy derivatives. This is because what drives PGA synthesis is not the soybean itself, but that infamous *Bacillus subtilis* fermentation process.

Fermented soybean products are a traditional Asian ingredient. Will globalization and the growing appeal of Japanese cuisine cause this kind of allergy to crop up in the United States? Only time will tell.

In conclusion:
Dear surfers of every nation,
You must banish natto from your diet—this is an
    obligation.
If you don't, *Bacillus subtilis* will gladly accept your
    invitation
And punish you with an allergy without the slightest
    hesitation.

Caviar—the diamonds of the sea?

I wanted to find just the right quotation to introduce this next section and chose the words of actor José Arthur: "The day the sturgeons learn the cost of caviar, they will become pretentious."

One does have to admit that the cost of this coveted luxury product is rather prohibitive. Who in the world would imagine that this delicate little snack could also be the source of severe allergic reactions? And yet, according to the medical literature, this is very much the case.

Beluga caviar—not as great as everyone says

Here's a real-life example that was published in 2002: on three separate occasions, a fifty-eight-year-old man quickly developed symptoms of anaphylaxis after ingesting beluga caviar. Strangely, he remembered eating it without any symptoms two years before (this was most likely when sensitization took place). When his case was first reported, the allergen had not yet been identified with any certainty, but researchers were already hypothesizing that vitellogenin was involved.*

Another man, age fifty-nine, had an allergic reaction to another protein—so far unidentified—that is also present in beluga eggs. He said he ingested a teaspoon of caviar and almost immediately felt severe anaphylactic symptoms. Upon arrival at the emergency room, he was hospitalized and monitored after the episode. Allergy testing analyzed his body's response to

---

* We will talk about this later; see page 75.

various fish and chicken eggs, but only one came back positive: beluga caviar.

An invisible allergen

A forty-eight-year-old luxury product buyer whose case is described in an article from July 2019 had an equally frightening experience. At a friend's house for dinner, the following items were on the menu: beluga caviar, foie gras, quail eggs, and blinis—all washed down with a sprinkling of champagne. Within minutes her ears started itching, she felt nauseated and faint, and her face and throat became swollen. The following year, she visited multiple caviar packaging plants without experiencing any symptoms. Already aware of her moderately severe asthma, she nevertheless decided to consult an allergist about the strange episode. All of the skin prick tests were negative except for two: oscietra caviar and imperial caviar. Her next round of visits to caviar production sites were more "complicated." She experienced respiratory symptoms that had been previously nonexistent in the very same situations, and her face also started itching. When she and her doctor finally got to the bottom of things, the invisible culprits turned out to be airborne beluga egg allergens. Since then she has carried an inhaler and an auto-injector with her at all times. The article explains that allergens from other fish eggs are very often found in beluga caviar. For this reason, people allergic to any kind of fish eggs should avoid consuming similar products.

Whether it's something in everyone's kitchen
Or if it costs the same as a new home addition
Foods contain allergens—yes, it bears repetition.
Never assume you can rule something out—pick up the
    phone and call your physician.
If you're showing symptoms
Don't twiddle your thumbs.
Keep a list of what was in your meal
So your allergist won't have to reinvent the wheel
To find out which allergen is causing such a stir.
Remember—the cost of what's on the table simply doesn't
    matter!

Dangerous dewdrops

"A rose, she too hath lived as long as live the roses, the space of one brief morn," François de Malherbe writes in his "Consolation Poem."[*]

Like the subject of the poem, a man from Güneykent in the Isparta region of Turkey came close to living his last morning, too. I will let you be the judge, but to my mind his story proves just how vitally important allergic investigation is, especially in a case such as this one where the trigger is absolutely impossible to identify early on. Here is what happened to him.

The main character in this account is a forty-seven-year-old asthmatic and former smoker, a chauffeur by trade, who is also allergic to various pollens and dust mites. For twenty years he has been suffering from chronic rhinitis with sneezing and a runny nose every day. His allergies get worse in the spring

---

[*]   Translation by Henry Wadsworth Longfellow.

during pollination, and in the past he has developed contact eczema after handling flowers, roses in particular. Sometimes when he eats honey his lips will swell and he has difficulty swallowing, but he has never paid this much attention.

For whatever reason, he has made a habit of waking at dawn and drinking a few dewdrops collected from rose petals. One morning, though, nothing goes as planned. Within thirty minutes, he is showing signs of anaphylactic shock. What could possibly be causing this? Solving this mystery will require an extensive investigation, and testing begins once the man has received proper medical treatment. Believe it or not, the tests reveal that his body was reacting to rose pollen that had dissolved in the dewdrops.

When it comes to allergies
Remember this rule, if you please:
Never, ever, in your wildest dreams
Rule out an allergen—the right diagnosis isn't always
   what it seems!

Note

Turkey, Morocco, Bulgaria, and China are the world's major rose producers. Roses in the Isparta region bloom from mid-May to mid-June and many people in the area depend on these flowers and related products like rose oil, jellies, and flavored desserts for their livelihoods. Every morning, the rose petals are plucked from the plants by hand before the sun can dry them out and cause the rose oil to evaporate. Then the petals are transported in baskets to a factory. Rhinitis and asthma resulting from contact with rose pollen have been reported, and this represents a public health problem for the people living in this region.

When beer makes your body itch

The introduction to these next few paragraphs dedicated to beer allergies was handed to me on a silver platter. While I was writing this book, my friend Christiane sent me a hilarious Mexican newspaper article—you'll see why I couldn't pass up the opportunity to include it somewhere in this section. I knew immediately that it was the perfect way to introduce this new topic.

The story is about a Mexican couple. The husband is obviously an alcoholic and drinks so much beer that one day his wife can't take it anymore. An insane idea takes root in this woman's mind: she decides to mix the beer with a laxative—in this case, a skillful combination of castor oil and prune juice.

She starts handing him his cans already opened—after garnishing them with a little something extra, of course. Amazed that she's being so magnanimous, her husband can't believe his good luck. Meanwhile, his wife is hoping that the symptoms he is about to experience will be mistaken for a beer allergy. As expected, her husband starts having terrible abdominal pain and diarrhea that sends him running to the bathroom—but he doesn't stop drinking the "new" beer!

You probably found this anecdote amusing, but there is one minor detail you should know. The alcoholic husband ended up in the emergency room with severe dehydration and his wife was taken to court for attempted homicide. These events were reported in the Mexican newspaper *Vanguardia*.

Those nasty LTPs

Despite that story's less than happy ending, it is still a relatively innocent case when one knows the truth about IgE-mediated beer allergy. Although rare, it certainly exists.

Yes, it's true. Drinking a pint is not necessarily synonymous with a good time. After a few sips, individuals with this allergy experience skin reactions (hives), swelling of the lips and throat, and difficulty breathing. These unusual symptoms should not be dismissed and are evidence of an allergy. The culprit protein is none other than lipid transfer protein, or LTP. Other allergens are sometimes involved, but not as frequently. We will look at those more closely later.

Note

LTPs defend plants against bacteria, fungi, and viruses. Their molecular structure keeps them from breaking down even at high temperatures (thermoresistance) and they can also withstand digestion, which may be why they provoke such severe allergic reactions.

Most people know how to order a beer, but do we actually know what's in it?

Let's take a quick look at the list of ingredients. It's a heady mix of:

• Malted barley, which is made by soaking and heating the grain. Other grains like rice, corn, and sorghum can also be used.

- Hops, which gives beer its bitterness.
- Brewer's yeast like *Saccharomyces cerevisiae* or *Saccharomyces carlsbergensis* for fermentation.

Now that we've covered this basic information, let's dive into this subject with a discussion of the frustrations experienced by a forty-five-year-old man in 2012. He is asthmatic, allergic to cats, grass pollen, and *Alternaria* mold, and every time he drinks beer he has difficulty breathing and becomes covered in hives. Worried, he makes an appointment with a specialist. The doctor conducts an in-depth interview and the patient undergoes skin prick tests for thirty-six different brands of beer. Thirty of them appear positive. Next up is a beer provocation test (like an oral food challenge) for the six brands that did not cause a reaction. This test takes place over several days, and the initial dose of 50 ml is increased daily until the patient reaches 500 ml. From an allergy standpoint, the patient tolerates the tests extremely well . . . but he is certainly not in any condition to get behind the wheel. Remember, this alcohol consumption was for diagnostic purposes, and alcohol abuse is dangerous for your health!

In this instance, the protein responsible for the allergy is not hops, but rather corn LTP. In some countries, corn is used to give beer a particular flavor. Interestingly, this man regularly eats polenta and popcorn without any unusual symptoms.

Note

A word of warning: Some restaurants add a teaspoon of beer to their vinaigrette without informing customers. Also remember that pancake and waffle batter may contain beer.

In another case published in 2019 in the *British Medical Journal*, a thirty-two-year-old man develops symptoms of anaphylaxis a few minutes after consuming a Franziskaner beer. No other alcoholic beverage provokes the same reaction in his body. He consults a specialist for allergy tests that are positive for wheat, barley, peach, and nine other beer brands. The culprits in this story are, once again, LTPs in the grain used to make the brew.

Where is it brewed?

When an allergist is trying to identify the beer allergen causing their patient's symptoms, they need to know what is in the beer, of course, but knowing the country where the beer is brewed is equally important information. In China, for example, out of twenty beer-allergic participants in a medical survey who agreed to undergo testing with various grains and yeasts, fifteen were positive for sorghum and sorghum malt. After beer provocation tests, hives and rashes were observed during the two hours following beer ingestion. While other participants were positive for hops, barley, and yeast, it is safe to assume that in China, sorghum—which is often used there to make beer—is the predominant allergen and the one most often responsible for allergic reactions.

Barley is used in beer to enhance and stabilize foam. Unlike in the sorghum example above, it's those villainous little barley LTPs that cause allergic reactions to malted barley, barley-based beer, or barley malt miso.

When the lips get involved

If someone is truly unlucky, he or she might be allergic to several different alcohols, not because of the grains they contain but because of other allergens like yeast.

> Other yeasts in addition to *Saccharomyces cerevisiae* are sometimes used in fermentation. These include *Saccharomyces pastorianus*, *Brettanomyces sp.*, and *Torulaspora delbrueckii*. The choice of yeast is dictated by whether the beer is dark or light and where it is brewed. Wines and hard ciders are fermented with different variants of *Saccharomyces cerevisiae*.

One young man, age nineteen, had the same sour experience every time he consumed beer, hard cider, wine, or champagne. Tasting a craft beer made with local ingredients triggered the most severe symptoms of all. His nose felt congested, his lungs "whistled," his skin was covered in hives, and he had trouble swallowing. He said he had no problem drinking gin and vodka, but whenever he ate a banana he would often get an itchy throat. He knew he was allergic to pollen and had a history of moderate eczema. After allergy testing, he discovered that he was also sensitive to a variety of molds. The specialist's conclusion was clear: this mold allergy was causing his body to react to yeast and alcoholic drinks containing it. He was told to avoid any and all foods that may contain these things. Since his reaction to wine and hard cider was most likely due to the yeasts they contain, he could continue eating apples and grapes without experiencing symptoms.

> If you suspect an allergy to beer
> Just stay calm and keep your thinking clear.
> Think about what the problem ingredient might be
> And in this way avoid a tragedy!

Against your skin

Don't let that heading fool you; I promise we're still talking about allergies! Most people think that eating an allergy-causing food is the only real way to trigger a food-related reaction, but this is not the case. There are other, more surprising situations that can provoke the same reactions, and being aware of them can save allergy-sufferers a significant amount of hassle. So let's discuss this other group of food allergy reactions where the allergen does not enter the body through the mouth, but through the skin.

The problem is in the peel . . .

In an article published in *The Sun* in January 2020, obstetrician-gynecologist Dr. Diana Gill issued a warning to all men who choose to pleasure themselves by masturbating into a banana peel. Yes, that is what I wrote. As surprising and perplexing as it sounds, this unconventional method is becoming more and more popular. The sensation these men are going for is supposedly similar to the experience of receiving oral sex.

According to online testimonials, banana peels also happen to be a "great lubricant."

One would hope that none of these banana peel enthusiasts are allergic to latex or bananas, because if they are, the doctor explains, they will not obtain the ecstasy they are looking for and instead risk developing hives, a swollen penis, and even anaphylaxis.

Note

Remember that latex cross-reactivities exist with chestnuts and exotic foods like banana, kiwi, and avocado. . . .

Direct contact between a food allergen and a person's skin can trigger violent and even fatal reactions. It is so important that people realize this so that events like those I am about to describe can be avoided.

Schoolboy tragedy

A thirteen-year-old boy of Indian origin living in England was known to be allergic to a variety of foods: wheat, peanut, cashew, cow's milk, egg, and walnut. He had already suffered several episodes of anaphylaxis linked to wheat consumption. As if this weren't bad enough, he also had asthma, eczema, and seasonal rhinitis. In 2017, one of his classmates threw a piece of cheese down his shirt. After just a few minutes, the poor boy started feeling very sick. He scratched the skin on his back until it bled. He pulled off his shirt. His breathing became labored and irregular. He was having an asthma attack, signaling the onset of anaphylaxis. Respiratory distress kicked in, but his inhaler had no effect. School personnel called an ambulance, but the epinephrine injection thirteen minutes later did nothing—unfortunately, the auto-injector had been expired for eleven months! The child's symptoms continued getting worse and he lost consciousness. The ambulance arrived around ten minutes later. The young boy was already in a coma and the ambulance team could not detect a pulse. He was transported directly to intensive care, but in spite of the efforts made to resuscitate him, he never regained consciousness and died almost two weeks later. His brain had sustained too much damage during the cardiac arrest.

This real example of a severe reaction from skin contact with a food allergen was not published in a medical journal until three years later, in January 2020. The article concludes that this is "the first documented case of fatal anaphylaxis potentially due to cutaneous exposure to a food allergen, in the absence of oral exposure." What could have been considered a joke between two classmates ended badly, and this tragedy led to charges of involuntary homicide. The coroner said the other student's action was "a childish and thoughtless act but was not calculated to cause serious harm." The charges have since been dropped, but many would categorize what happened as an example of the harassment and intimidation targeting people with food allergies that is becoming more and more widespread.

What does Peter Rabbit have to do with this?

When the animated film *Peter Rabbit* was released in 2018, it was met with harsh criticism from viewers around the world concerned about what they termed "allergy bullying." One scene in particular had the American allergy organization Kids with Food Allergies immediately up in arms, and Australia's Global Anaphylaxis Awareness and Inclusivity organized an online petition demanding that the film be pulled from theaters. In the United Kingdom, the reaction from Allergy UK president Carla Jones was equally damning. The French organization AFPRAL* also discussed the film in its quarterly review.

The scene in question may appear innocent, but families with allergies feel differently. Tom McGregor, Peter Rabbit's archenemy, happens to be allergic to blackberries. War breaks out between the rabbits and Tom, the man who has taken over "their land," and the menacing animals threaten to throw blackberries at him to make him sick. Which is precisely what they proceed to do. They bombard him with berries until they manage to get one in his mouth and the gardener goes into anaphylactic shock. He falls to his knees. Before he passes out he manages to give himself a shot of epinephrine. He quickly regains consciousness, stands up, and the battle continues.

People with allergies have every reason to find this scene painful to watch. They know just how deadly a food allergy can be. After the film's release, the hashtag #BoycottPeterRabbit

---

* Association française pour la prévention des allergies (French Association for the Prevention of Allergies).

appeared on a well-known social media platform whose symbol is a blue bird. The controversy continued to surge, and the film director, Will Gluck, along with Sony Pictures apologized in a statement acknowledging that the film "should not have made light of" food allergies.

Blackberry allergy is extremely rare and—unlike the other allergies we have discussed in this section—research today suggests it is triggered by ingesting blackberries, not via skin contact. The allergen responsible has not been identified, but people with allergies to other fruits in the Rosaceae family (apple, apricot, etc.) may also react to blackberries. A forty-five-year-old man had an anaphylactic reaction after eating blackberries, even though he had been experiencing mild reactions to blackberries, raspberries, and peanuts for twenty-five years. In 2017, though, several English medical journals described a very different case: little Nainika Tikoo was a nine-year-old girl with asthma living near London. She was allergic to milk, soy, and eggs, and her father would happily make her allergy-friendly pancakes. One day she asked him to add blackberries, a fruit she had never tried before. After one bite, she had a severe allergic reaction and lost consciousness. Her parents called an ambulance and her father quickly injected her with epinephrine, but the intensity of her reaction sent her into cardiac arrest. She was placed on advanced life support and the doctors informed her loved ones that her brain had suffered irreversible damage. The child died five days later. In her memory, her parents created a foundation in her name with a JustGiving page. Their goal is to raise money to bring allergy awareness to the larger public and to finance allergy research.

What about cow's milk protein?

Believe it or not, a few non-fatal cases of skin-induced reactions to cow's milk protein have been reported. A baby boy with this allergy had a violent reaction after his skin came into contact with a body cream containing this protein. Luckily, his life was saved by an injection of epinephrine. A young woman with the same allergy experienced anaphylactic symptoms during a boxing class due to the unsuspected presence of cow's milk protein in her new pair of boxing gloves.

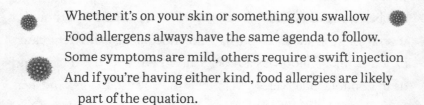

Whether it's on your skin or something you swallow
Food allergens always have the same agenda to follow.
Some symptoms are mild, others require a swift injection
And if you're having either kind, food allergies are likely
part of the equation.

A joint and a peach . . .

Yes, I do mean that kind of joint—we're going to be talking about "pot," "Mary Jane," cannabis, call it whatever you like. So what's the connection between a wholesome fruit and this illicit substance? You are in for a surprise.

In our first case, a young man we'll call Matthew smokes hashish two or three nights a week. Why? He says it helps him sleep better. In addition to this, he'll also puff on a joint at a party with friends once in a while. He does not smoke cigarettes and grows small cannabis plants in his apartment for his own use. For some time, though, he's been bothered by a case of rhinitis he can't seem to shake. But that's certainly not enough to stop him. He continues smoking hashish regularly and marijuana occasionally. One day, Matthew is sitting at dinner with his family and decides to eat a peach for dessert that has been washed but not peeled. Suddenly his life is turned upside down. A few minutes go by and his palms suddenly start itching. His lips double in size, he has difficulty swallowing, and he feels extremely ill. His family is sure he's going into anaphylactic shock. Horrified, they call for an ambulance and one arrives shortly after. A rapid injection of epinephrine fortunately saves his life. After several hours of monitoring at the hospital, Matthew returns home. A few months later, an allergy test reveals that the peach was indeed the culprit. His body had reacted to a protein in the LTP family that causes severe allergic reactions. Then the allergist asks the big question: "Do you use cannabis?" Why is that relevant? There's a very simple reason, and it's called cannabis-fruit and vegetable syndrome (or cannabis allergy).

In 2009, there were an estimated 125 to 203 million occasional or regular cannabis users between the ages of fifteen and sixty-four around the world. And, since the substance in question is largely prohibited in many places, this number is likely an underestimation.

Be careful, ladies and gentlemen

Cannabis sativa is a flowering plant from the Cannabaceae family. Its pollen grains measure 23–28 μm in diameter and are carried on the wind (cannabis is anemophilous, or wind pollinated) from late summer to early fall. The majority of it grows in cultivation areas located in central India, southern Europe, Pakistan, and the United States, but people also grow it in its wild state for personal use.

A few years ago, France's National Network for Aerobiological Surveillance (RNSA) collected data showing the presence of cannabis pollen in Aix-en-Provence, Grenoble, Bourgoin, Mâcon, Roussillon, and Strasbourg between late July and late August. Later that year, the sensors detected the same pollen in Ajaccio, Corsica.

One of the substances in cannabis, delta-9-tetrahydrocannabinol (THC), is known for being a particularly potent psychoactive compound. It can be smoked or chewed in the form of marijuana (dried flowers containing 25 percent THC), or hashish (dried resin, 10–30 percent THC). Sometimes it is also added to foods as a highly concentrated oil (between 60 and 80 percent THC). In the United States, it is legal to grow hemp for industrial use as long as it conforms to regulatory framework set by the USDA in the 2018 Farm Bill.

Let's briefly review the harmful side effects linked to "recreational" cannabis use. These include dry mouth, pupil dilation (a classic), tremors, and increased heart rate. Then there are the problems with concentration and memory. Cannabis smoke also contains seven times more tar and carbon monoxide than tobacco smoke, and this toxic effect is multiplied when it is smoked with a water pipe.

Cannabis allergies

The first description of an allergic reaction to cannabis was published in 1971. The case involved a twenty-nine-year-old female who was "forced" to give up using marijuana to avoid the risk of a potentially deadly anaphylactic reaction. In 2012, a medical team studied fifteen marijuana users who displayed allergy symptoms like rhinitis, conjunctivitis, sinusitis, periorbital edema, wheezing, and swelling of the throat after inhaling cannabis smoke. Other symptoms were also mentioned, including swelling of the uvula lasting several hours or even days.

Another health hazard, aspergillus mold, is a common cannabis contaminant that can lead to the development of severe asthma in the long term. Last, but certainly not least, the consumption of cannabis seeds, either alone or infused in tea, can cause anaphylaxis.

Even more troubling than the symptoms mentioned above is the negative effect cannabis smoke has on people around the user who are not smoking the drug. An article from November 2018 describes the case of a six-year-old with asthma whose condition is getting worse despite aggressive treatment. An extensive interview with an allergy specialist reveals that members of his family, including his maternal grandmother, are regular cannabis users. What's more, his grandma admits to having a few "issues" including hives when she uses it. Just to be sure, she and her grandson undergo a series of tests that confirm a true allergy to cannabis.* The little boy's asthma improves almost immediately once he is no longer exposed to secondhand cannabis smoke.

Cross-reactivities

The fact that we are seeing so many severe food allergy reactions among cannabis users is, in my opinion, something worth exploring further here and in the allergy field. Take the case of a twenty-eight-year-old cannabis user who experiences itching, rhinitis, and swollen eyelids every time he smokes. He also develops food allergies to peaches, apples, almonds, eggplants, and chestnuts. Certain foods—tomato, bell pepper, and fig—trigger symptoms so severe they are considered anaphylactic.

The allergen responsible for this young man's health problems is an LTP called Can s 3 that is heat-resistant and remains intact throughout its journey along the digestive tract, which explains why the food allergy reactions are so sudden and severe (anaphylaxis, generalized hives, asthma attacks). People who have been sensitized to Can s 3 through cannabis use risk having a reaction to peaches, apples, cherries, hazelnuts, tomatoes (raw or cooked), and certain citrus fruits like grapefruit and oranges. Beer, wine, latex, and tobacco are also potentially cross-reactive with cannabis.

---

* An immediate IgE-mediated allergy that is unrelated to cross-reactivity.

If you happen to be smoking weed
Pause for a moment and take heed.
Sudden swelling, cough, or hives?
It could be an allergy—man alive!
As soon as these symptoms come to be
At once your doctor, you'd better see
This also means you'll have to kick your habit
If you don't want these problems multiplying like rabbits.
And one more thing before I go:
Legally speaking, it's usually a no-no.

Dangerous inhalations

Earlier we talked about one lesser-known pathway for food allergens entering the body—the skin—but the possibilities don't stop there: food allergens can also be *inhaled*. The two cases I am about to share prove that for people with food allergies, danger can indeed be everywhere, even when we least expect it. The first story takes place in someone's personal life and the second in a work context.

When the truth comes to light

A young woman in her twenties with eczema and asthma decides to consult a specialist. She is diagnosed with allergies to pollen, cats, and eggs. During the oral food challenge for egg, she starts having significant difficulty breathing after ingesting 100 mg in the form of a powder. She is told to avoid eggs in her diet and her skin improves as a result. Fifteen months later, an old sixteenth-century cathedral near her home is under renovation. She inhales dust from the construction site and this provokes a violent asthma attack. An in-depth investigation is conducted to understand her reaction, and after extensive research, one of the doctors has an idea. As far back as Ancient Rome, adding egg to sealants was commonplace and helped protect stone buildings. If the patina of the old walls contains egg proteins, maybe that's what triggered this young woman's allergy. The next round of research leaves no room for doubt: there are indeed egg proteins in the old sealant, and the level of egg white-specific IgE antibodies in the young woman's system is off the charts at 1,000 ku/l.[*]

Note

The doctors on this case put forward several hypotheses and ultimately found the solution to the puzzle in an archaeological review. The article that changed everything had been written to provide direct evidence for the practice of animal husbandry and dairy production on the Atlantic coast of Scotland 2,500 years ago during the Iron Age, namely the presence of milk proteins in prehistoric vessels. This publication was a breakthrough in the allergists' investigation and led to the allergen's discovery.

Walnuts hiding in the dust . . .

In 2017, a man in his thirties with tree nut allergies died tragically while on the job. He was supposed to conduct air quality testing at a fire station that was under renovation. The walls of the building had recently been stripped using a sandblasting product made with walnut shells. Twenty minutes after he

---

[*]   Normal values are below 0.1 ku/l.

arrived, he started having difficulty breathing and crumpled to the ground outside the building. His family suspected that he had inhaled nut allergens in the air that caused his anaphylaxis. The construction company had chosen this particular sandblasting product as an eco-friendly alternative to silica, which can damage the lungs.

No matter where you are—in your house, at school, in a restaurant, on a flight, in a convenience store—you can almost always find a food allergen lurking somewhere. They may be in something as seemingly insignificant as a smell or cooking vapors, but once these allergens are inhaled by people already sensitized to them, they trigger explosive symptoms like hives, swelling, rhino-conjunctivitis, asthma attacks, and even anaphylaxis. Wheat flour, shellfish, soy, peanuts, fish, eggs, and milk top the list of major offenders. Who could have ever imagined that even walls could be dangerous?

Trouble in the air

Typically, food allergy reactions caused by inhalation occur in individuals who have already been sensitized to the food allergen after ingesting it at an earlier date. This pattern appears in quite a number of published cases, including those of an eleven-year-old who exhibited anaphylactic symptoms while his mother was cooking rice and a woman with cow's milk protein allergy who went into anaphylactic shock after walking through a milk storage area in a barn. A more recent publication reports that a young boy allergic to peanuts had a severe reaction while standing next to a birdcage where peanuts were present.

I use the word "typically" because sensitization can just as easily take place as a result of inhaling a food allergen. This can lead to an allergic reaction when the allergen is later ingested for the first time. Simply put, the inhalation sensitizes without creating a reaction, then the ingestion of the food allergen causes the reaction—the exact opposite of the cases I described in the paragraph above! To illustrate this, let's look at the case of six bakery workers. They all suffered from rhino-conjunctivitis and four of them also had asthma. Doctors determined that the cause of their symptoms was exposure to airborne egg proteins. Half of the group later developed allergy symptoms after egg ingestion, but these were observed *after* the development of respiratory allergy symptoms (from inhalation), not at the same time. I must also mention the story of a sixty-year-old woman who worked as a home health aide and regularly inhaled psyllium powder while preparing laxatives for her patients. She later had an anaphylactic reaction while eating a mixture of grains that contained psyllium.

As an allergist I curse those walls—
The ones hiding food allergens in their depths
Launching surprise attacks on allergy sufferers—the gall!
And leading some to an untimely death.
With this in mind, I'll say again:
To avoid bad luck you'll need vigilance times ten.
And if you feel like you need epinephrine
Don't hesitate for a second—give yourself that injection!

A twenty-four-carat allergy

When a person is allergic to other metals like nickel, they are very often advised to choose jewelry made from eighteen- or twenty-four-carat gold. Unfortunately, sometimes the body plays tricks on us and has a negative reaction to gold salts.

The first instances of this interesting phenomenon were described in 1990. However, the validity of the skin tests that were used in several of the reported cases is debatable. As a result, overdiagnosis is a distinct possibility.

When a trip to the dentist proves very revealing

We'll begin with the story of a thirty-six-year-old woman whose allergy problem was reported in the *Revue française d'allergologie* (RFA) in 2008. This woman had been selling jewelry for six years when she began noticing eczema on her hands that persisted for several months. Mysteriously, the skin lesions disappeared when she was on maternity leave. Her physician suspected something job-related. Regrettably, her allergy tests at the time were inconclusive and couldn't point to any real cause for her reaction. A few months later, apparently, she developed "petechial" lesions inside her mouth. This discovery led her dentist to send her back to an allergist. A new round of testing began, and this time included what is called a dental battery, which tests for gold sodium thiosulfate (GST) among other things. This allergen is a marker of gold allergies and was her only positive test result. This same test was positive again one month later, even after the patient had left her job in the jewelry business.

Since the positive GST test correlated with the timeline of her clinical history, she was diagnosed with a gold allergy.

Where else does gold slip in?

The medical literature contains a range of reported gold allergy symptoms including eczema on the earlobes, neck, or wrist after wearing gold jewelry. Gold has also been observed to cause allergy-related issues in dental crowns and implants; while it has been gradually replaced by resin and other materials, these days this metal can still be found adorning the mouths of elderly individuals and certain rap artists.

Wearing gold jewelry represents one level of exposure, but we should keep in mind the amount of contact with this metal that jewelers, dental technicians, and cutlers have to deal with on a daily basis. The same is true for people who handle printed circuit boards, bind gold-embossed books, or restore paintings and other decorative objects. Electroplaters, too, often report having eczema on their fingers and eyelids. Electroplaters? I confess that I had to Google this, but an electroplater is a professional who uses an electrochemical process to coat objects with a thin layer of metal.

In the medical domain, gold salts are used to treat diseases like rheumatoid arthritis, and cardiologists place gold-plated stents to improve angina symptoms.

As doctors, we cannot help but be interested in the hubbub surrounding the new gastronomic trend of decorating everything from steak to chocolate to baked goods with pieces of edible twenty-four-carat gold leaf. Will we eventually see food allergies triggered by the ingestion of this metal? All we can do is wait to find out.

Studies performed in the 2000s support the hypothesis that women are more commonly affected by this allergy than men. This is most likely because women tend to have more piercings and wear gold jewelry more often, which may facilitate sensitization.

In the jewelry business, other metals are often added to gold to make an alloy. This gives the gold extra durability, resistance to corrosion, and can also change the color of the gold if desired. Nickel, for example, gives it a pale yellow or white color (white gold), and copper gives gold a reddish tint. People who are allergic to gold may also be allergic to other metals in these alloys.

> If at times gold becomes your enemy
> And it appears to be the only thing tarnishing your beauty
> Those red patches on your skin
> Are telling you to find an allergist who'll fit you in!
> To prevent the blossoming of another rash,
> You'll have to nip this in the bud and choose another
>   metal—fast.

Is there an allergen on the plane?

They've been planning this trip for months. Five girlfriends have decided to take off to another country (somewhere sunny in southern Spain, as it happens) without their significant others. The young women are planning to stay with an old friend who has been living in Spain for a few years, and they already know their schedule: lazy mornings, lounging on the beach, partying, and of course, shopping. Everything has been prepared down to the smallest detail. Lisa, Margot, Laura, and Patricia even managed to convince Sarah to come with them. She's a little worried about leaving home, and even though she always has her emergency epinephrine nearby, her peanut allergy does limit her ability to travel somewhat. Her last anaphylactic episode was three years ago, and the memory of it is still permanently etched in her mind. Nevertheless, she is determined to go on this dream vacation. After a consultation with her allergist to go over everything, Sarah contacts the airline. It's important for her to find out what ingredients their in-flight meals will contain. She has a prescription written in English and Spanish in her bag with her emergency medication, and she now feels relaxed about the trip. Without a care in the world, the five ladies board the plane. The beginning of the flight goes off without a hitch—then a passenger sitting not far from Sarah pulls out a bag of salted peanuts and starts eating them. Sarah is highly reactive to this food and immediately starts having trouble breathing. Her face becomes covered in hives and her lips swell. She knows the symptoms all too well. Luckily, her auto-injector pen is in her carry-on. One of her friends gives her an injection followed by a second shot a few minutes later because the anaphylaxis symptoms are so severe. The pilot is informed about what is happening and when the plane lands a few minutes later, Sarah is quickly taken to be hospitalized for monitoring. The rest of the vacation goes as planned.

A high-risk journey

The catastrophic scenario above is based on real events. In 2018 alone, a number of articles reported the disastrous consequences of food allergy reactions observed in an air travel context. When the allergic reaction occurs in an enclosed space like the cabin, the stories in these articles sometimes end in tragedy. It's not hard to understand why—unless your name is Clark Kent there is simply no way to exit a plane in midair. Severe anaphylaxis during a flight affects around 1 percent of people with food allergies. Tree nuts and peanuts are the major allergens responsible. A 2002 study of 3,704 air travelers with allergies found that 41 of them had problems during a flight. Half of them were able to handle the allergy attack on their own without a problem. Twelve travelers asked for help from the flight crew. Six severe reactions led to planes being rerouted for emergency landings.

There are many things that can trigger a food allergy inside an airplane. The ventilation system, for one thing, contributes to the dispersal of airborne allergenic particles. Even if only twenty-five passengers each open a bag of peanuts at the same time, in a closed environment like the plane cabin that's enough to expose all of the other passengers to secondary inhalation of allergenic proteins. Serving a snack like peanut-flavored puffs only makes it easier for the allergen to diffuse throughout the air in the cabin. Deposits of these same allergens on tray tables or seats is another possibility that people with allergies should be prepared for. A young Australian woman with a peanut allergy encountered this issue in 2018 and even posted a photo of her swollen face on Facebook—her reaction started shortly after she boarded the plane!

Food labels—whether the items are offered during a flight or purchased before boarding—should always be examined closely, even when it seems unnecessary. A story reported in the *Guardian* in 2018 sadly proves this point. Fifteen-year-old Natasha, along with her father and a friend, was flying from London to Nice on a British Airways flight. She bought a premade sandwich at an airport kiosk that contained bread, artichoke, olives, and tapenade. Knowing she was allergic to several foods including sesame seeds, she and her father checked the label twice instead of once. But even that proved insufficient because the young girl collapsed during the flight after eating the sandwich. An emergency injection of epinephrine and resuscitation efforts were unable to subdue the effects of extreme shock, and Natasha died within hours. Her mother investigated and discovered that the bread did indeed contain sesame, but it was not listed on the label.

Caution is the mother of safety

Planes can be dangerous places for people with all kinds of food allergies, especially if the flight is several hours long. Travelers with allergies (and airlines!) would be wise to take certain precautions before takeoff.

Consulting your allergist before you leave should be a priority, especially if you are traveling abroad. He or she will make sure your allergy action plan is up to date and write you any prescriptions you may need. Medications should be written using the international nonproprietary name (INN) or generic name to make them easier to identify if you are in a foreign country. Your emergency medications and these medical recommendations should be easy to access in your carry-on luggage. They should never be in your checked bags!

It is also a good idea to inform the airline about your allergy as soon as you book your ticket. On the day of your flight, talk to the crew about your allergies when you board the plane. Use these conversations as an opportunity to find out exactly what food will be served during the in-flight meal.

Some companies have tried developing allergen-free "buffer zones" for travelers with food allergies, but this has not been very successful. Other airlines prohibit the sale of peanuts during the flight but allow passengers to eat them if they purchased the peanuts before takeoff.

Allergies (and not just food allergies) are the seventh leading cause of in-flight medical problems. They are also responsible for 4 percent of emergencies during commercial flights. Airline companies that are aware of these risks take certain measures by maintaining an emergency medical kit that ideally contains a blood pressure monitor, stethoscope, epinephrine auto-injector, inhaler, and antihistamine and steroid treatments in pill and injectable form. But how can you be sure this will be the case for every flight you take? It's best to check before flying and make sure not to forget your own medications.

You and your allergies are free to fly off to another country
As long as your epinephrine is nearby and stored securely.
Never let your doctor's note out of your sight
That way if there's trouble, you'll still be all right.
If you carry your medication and take these precautions
I'm certain you'll be able to enjoy your vacation.

More fish egg problems

Their friends had invited them to come over for dinner three weeks ago and the couple is thrilled to be seeing them again. They haven't gotten together in so long; life, work, their kids, and a packed schedule don't always make getting together with friends an easy feat. But today is the day. The family pulls up to the house where their hosts are eagerly waiting. A marvelously laid table signals the wonderful evening ahead. Cocktails are served with bursts of laughter and lively conversation. The friends' long-awaited reunion is everything they hoped it would be. Appetizers of all kinds are on hand to accompany the champagne. The children, naturally, are drinking fruit juice. There are pistachios and peanuts, cherry tomatoes, savory breads, and tiny toasts topped with taramasalata, salmon roe, tapenade, and small slices of sausage. Everything is wonderful until Jonathan feels an itch. He starts coughing and furiously scratching his palms. His lips swell and he breaks out in hives all over his body. His wife, Jennifer, is very worried—she has never seen him like this. She knows he's allergic to dust mites, but the panic on her face makes it plain that she knows this is different. Jonathan has never been aware of any peanut or tree nut allergies, but his symptoms certainly resemble anaphylaxis. After the administration of an epinephrine injection, he is taken by ambulance to the hospital where he is monitored for twenty-four hours before returning home to his beloved wife.

This fictional account may sound far-fetched, but allergies to fish eggs other than caviar do exist, though they are rare. Salmon roe are first on the list of prime suspects.

The allergen that Jonathan reacted to is entirely unrelated to fish meat. The problem actually comes from a protein in the fish eggs called vitellogenin. Hold on to your hats: vitellogenin is a glycophospholipoprotein that females synthesize during their reproductive cycle. As the egg develops, vitellogenin is broken down into lipovitellin, phosvitin, and beta components and becomes a source of nutrients for the fish embryo.

Vitellogenin is also found in chicken eggs and the eggs of arthropods like dust mites. The allergic reaction I described was probably caused by group 14 allergens in dust mites that, like vitellogenin, are precursors to lipovitellin and phosvitin. How great is all this new vocabulary, right? Since these precursors are only somewhat similar in structure to vitellogenin, however, cross-reactivity is rare.

This unusual food allergy is encountered most often in Japan and in Scandinavian countries where people tend to consume large amounts of fish. Adults represent the majority of cases, but there have been reports of pediatric cases, as we are about to see. A thirteen-year-old boy with multiple allergies ingested *Oncorhynchus keta* (salmon eggs) during a meal and rapidly developed angioedema. Another child, a seven-year-old girl allergic to pistachios, complained of throat pain and swollen lips after eating salmon eggs. Five years later, she suffered an anaphylactic reaction after eating trout eggs, even though she had never reacted to them before. An atopic young man, age sixteen, ate toast topped with salmon eggs and thirty minutes later started feeling early symptoms of severe anaphylaxis. A twelve-year-old girl exhibited swollen lips and hives on her torso a few minutes after eating taramasalata made with cod eggs. Her doctor performed skin tests for cod and salmon eggs as well as fish meat. Only cod eggs came back positive. A supervised oral food challenge provoked swollen eyelids, conjunctivitis, and itching in the mouth. This child also tested positive for dust mite allergy.

Not sure where you'd encounter fish eggs? You'll just have to keep an eye out—but atop little pieces of toast at a cocktail party is a good place to start. Lumpfish eggs are a popular alternative to beluga caviar, so there's a good chance they'll be the ones you run into. Though naturally pale in color, they are often dyed with food coloring to make them more "attractive."

Fish eggs don't have to be from sturgeon
To kickstart your body's food allergy engine.
So keep them in mind if you have a reaction
To help your allergist determine the best course of action.

Tango that tingles

Young Maria is fascinated by South American culture and everything that goes with it—whether it's the music of Carlos Gardel, films by Carlos Saura, or *Last Tango in Paris*, she loves it all. It almost seems to be in her DNA. She recently decided to register for a ballroom dance class to learn the tango, and now nothing makes her happier than these weekly sessions. She learns quickly and finds herself in total osmosis with her partner, Ronald. When he travels for work, though, her teacher—the *muy caliente* Sebastian—steps in to lead. He is originally from Argentina but has adopted the United States as his home. His long jet-black hair is often tied back in a ponytail.

Over the past few months, Maria has noticed dry itchy red patches appear on her forehead. They eventually go away but always reappear after a few days. The young woman wonders why this skin problem has suddenly gotten worse in recent weeks, and she decides to ask an allergist. The doctor begins testing and quickly finds the guilty party: PPD (paraphenylenediamine), an ingredient in hair dyes. Remember this name, because you're going to hear it talked about a lot in this book! The specialist explains that Maria is experiencing a contact allergy "by proxy" (consort allergy), meaning she is reacting to a product on someone else's body. After thinking back to the eczema outbreaks and talking to friends and family, Maria finally figures it out. Sebastian, the handsome dark-haired dancer, is actually going gray and dyes his hair regularly. The dye he uses is found to contain the allergen Maria is reacting to. This explains why when she dances with Ronald, who is as blond as a field of wheat, her forehead always looks the same. When he's absent, the trouble starts . . . and all because of her dance teacher's hair.

One of the most beautiful definitions of Latin dance I've heard comes from English television journalist Angela Rippon. She calls tango "the closest thing you'll find to a vertical expression of a horizontal desire." But when consort allergies get involved—as two other dance lovers discovered—it's a very different story.

I read about this ballroom dance teacher's unfortunate experience in a dermatology article published in 2010. The woman, age forty, develops eczema on her right hand, back, waist, and left foot. She regularly gives tango lessons and suspects that the dermatitis is related to the close physical contact that is part of this style of dance. She knows she is allergic to perfumes and deodorants and remembers a bubbly skin reaction on her left foot after applying ketoprofen gel a few years ago.

There are two other very important details in this story. The day before the eczema appeared, our "victim" used a tanning bed. One of her students also uses the very same ketoprofen gel she once had a reaction to. This means that his hands deposited the allergens onto his teacher's skin while they were dancing together. The allergen that is transferred onto the teacher's skin also managed to penetrate her clothing. This may have been facilitated by the previous tanning-bed session, the teacher's clothing rubbing against her skin during the dance, or sweating.

Our second case is more recent, and the victim of this odd turn of events is a fifty-three-year-old man. For almost three years, he has been experiencing eczema-like lesions on his right temple. He has no known allergies. The red patches refuse to go away and he eventually consults an expert. The first round of testing shows a clear allergy to PPD. The allergist then asks him about his personal habits. He mentions that he was bitten by the tango bug a long time ago and that he has been dancing for many years. His tango partner, who is clearly quite a minx, wears makeup and (more importantly) dyes her hair with a product the dancer is allergic to. The close contact between the two—in this case dancing glued at the temple—combined with sweat made it easier for the allergen to come into contact with and penetrate the man's skin.

Over the past few years, men's cosmetics sales have gone through the roof, and any one of those moisturizers, anti-wrinkle creams, colognes, deodorants, or hair products could be the cause of a spouse's contact eczema. This is why these products should always be included in diagnostic testing to rule them out. I should also mention that the case of an allergy to ketoprofen gel is not as uncommon as it sounds. It is known to trigger contact allergies and is also widely used, making it a likely suspect in allergy investigations.

> The allergen in this case is here to spoil the romance
> Engraved in the steps of this Argentine dance.
> If your partner's touch seems to be twirling you into
>   contact allergies left and right
> An allergist's help and expertise will be able to shed some
>   light.

The strange allergic effect of the thirsty tick

Oscar is a carnivore, there's no doubt about that. Steak tartare, rare meat, beef carpaccio, nothing stops him. Among other physical activities, he enjoys walking with his girlfriend in the nearby forest. Recently, however, he has noticed that every time he eats red meat he breaks out in hives and feels itchy six to eight hours after the meal. He consults an allergist who understands exactly what the problem is by the end of the interview. He asks Oscar a question that seems to have little to do with why he made this appointment. As a matter of fact, yes, he had been bitten by a tick on his thigh a few months ago. He had been worried about Lyme disease and went to see his general practitioner, but once that was off the table he had completely forgotten about it. But now he'll remember it for the rest of his life—because he won't be able to eat red meat ever again! Let me explain to you why.

What connection could there possibly be between a tick bite and Oscar's reaction to meat? No connection at all, you might say. And besides, you might add, people seem more concerned about Lyme disease, anyway. While the second statement is true, a newly emerging food allergy called alpha-gal syndrome is proof that the allergist had every reason to wonder about his meat-loving patient's tick bite.

Ixodidae, more commonly known as ticks, develop and survive by feeding on blood from human and animal hosts as soon as they have hatched into larvae. They typically nest in areas of dense vegetation on the edges of forests and fields waiting for their prey in spring and early autumn. These distant (and disgusting) cousins of spiders and dust mites eagerly gorge them-selves on their host's blood, which sometimes means they can be infected by *Borrelia* bacteria contained in that blood. Ticks then transmit this infectious agent, which causes Lyme disease, to their next host in their saliva. As if this wasn't reason enough to dislike these bloodthirsty arachnids, recent studies confirm that this same tick saliva can play a major role in setting the stage for meat allergies by sensitizing the body to a carbohydrate prettily named galactose-alpha-1,3-galactose (alpha-gal).

Whereas most IgE-mediated food allergies are a reaction to a *protein* found in plant or animal tissues, alpha-gal syndrome is unique because in this case the allergy is to a *carbohydrate*. Allergists have been trying to solve this mystery ever since its first cases were discovered in Australia and the United States in 2009. Researchers quickly discovered that alpha-gal, which is only present in non-primate mammals, was behind many of the red meat allergies reported in areas where ticks are common. When someone is bitten by a tick and alpha-gal is transmitted in the tick's saliva, the body responds by manufacturing anti-al-pha-gal IgE antibodies. Repeated contact with alpha-gal through additional tick bites leads to sensitization, and symptoms of the developed allergy will appear when the carbohydrate is ingested in the form of red meat or organ meat.

Interestingly, people who have been sensitized to this curi-ous carbohydrate may also have a subsequent allergic reaction to a cancer drug called cetuximab that is used to treat meta-static colorectal cancer and epidermoid carcinoma of the neck.

Since cetuximab contains alpha-gal, a patient's levels of anti-alpha-gal IgE antibodies may need to be measured before it is administered the first time to avoid a serious allergic reaction. Individuals with alpha-gal syndrome should also be aware that alpha-gal is present in medical products like surgical implants and certain intravenous fluids containing animal gelatin.

Anyone who lives in a tick-infested area and enjoys eating red meat and organ meat—especially pig's kidneys—should pay close attention to the slightest sign of a food allergy reaction after they eat these foods. Another distinctive feature of alpha-gal syndrome is the unusually long delay between ingestion and the appearance of symptoms, so swelling, hives, and even anaphylaxis may not show up for three to eight hours after that juicy steak! I should also mention that alcohol consumption, NSAID use, or exercise after the meal can exacerbate the reaction.

Even though there is still much for the scientific community to learn about alpha-gal syndrome, if a patient is experiencing chronic hives, an allergy to red meat should always be investigated as a potential culprit.

Note

An altogether different meat-related allergy called pork-cat syndrome is linked to a protein called serum albumin and was given its somewhat peculiar name after researchers observed people with cat allergies (allergen Fel d 2) exhibiting hives, swelling, and anaphylactic symptoms after eating pork. Our understanding of this allergy has evolved and several studies have since confirmed that a potential cross-reactivity also exists with serum albumins found in cow's milk, cat and dog dander, and fish parvalbumin.

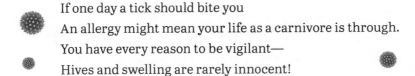

If one day a tick should bite you
An allergy might mean your life as a carnivore is through.
You have every reason to be vigilant—
Hives and swelling are rarely innocent!

Babies, milk, and cows . . . wow!

It could be said that cow's milk protein allergy has been known about for ages, but there are still so many errors in diagnosis that it's worth going over its unique characteristics.

"Got milk?" You may or may not remember those ads, but what we know for sure is that this nutritious drink (in the form of breastmilk or formula) is absolutely indispensable from the moment a baby is born. We also know that unfortunately for some of those babies, milk can become a real source of discomfort. Cow's milk protein allergy (CMPA) is, for many parents, a hell filled with questions and confusion. They find themselves wrongly accused of being overprotective, even though they are the ones making sure their children are sleeping and eating well. They are the ones who, after paying close attention to their baby, notice that something is definitely not right. *Why is my baby having diarrhea? Why is her stomach always so round? Why does he get so upset after his bottle? What about these never-ending bouts of hives and eczema?* These parents change the formula they're using and nothing is any better. Then one day, after an allergy test, the diagnosis arrives: their baby is allergic to cow's milk protein. Luckily, solutions do exist. Let's explore this allergy—one that to this day is all too often overlooked or misunderstood—so we can help young and old manage this problem. Fortunately, in most cases, this allergy "heals" itself spontaneously (50 percent of the time before the age of five, and 80 percent of the time by adolescence).

Milk is the foundation of every newborn's diet, and every mom makes the choice between breastfeeding and feeding with formula, which meets a baby's nutritional needs by aiming to resemble the composition of breastmilk as much as possible. There is, however, one important detail that should draw our attention: most of the time, formula is made with cow's milk, which means it contains the very proteins that can lead a baby to develop CMPA. But don't go thinking that breastfeeding eliminates this risk—infants can be sensitized to cow's milk proteins or other mammal milk proteins when the mother ingests dairy products and the proteins enter her breastmilk!

CMPA will usually appear within the first months of life or, occasionally, a little bit later. We'll look at a few examples and the various circumstances that lead to a cow's milk protein allergy diagnosis.

CMPA stories . . .
Such a pretty baby, but . . .
Born at full term, little Sarah has arrived in her new home after leaving her mother's comfortable belly just a few days ago. The new parents are completely over the moon and Sarah's grandparents are equally overjoyed. Both parents have allergies— Dad (Thierry) reacts every year to grass seed pollen and Mom

(Caroline) can't stand dust because of her dust mite allergy—and Grandma has had atopic eczema since childhood. Caroline has decided not to breastfeed and both parents are equally involved in preparing the baby's formula. They know exactly how much to give with each bottle, and everything goes well for the first few days. Total bliss, not a cloud in the sky. But then the sky darkens when their daughter starts vomiting each time she has a bottle. Soon Sarah is refusing to drink the formula. Her stomach is often swollen. She starts having foul-smelling diarrhea. The nights become more and more sleepless for the worried and exhausted parents. They change formula brands seven times but nothing helps. They try an antiregurgitation formula and thickening the liquid in the bottle, but the symptoms continue. Nothing changes. They are hopeless and at a loss. To make matters worse, the constant stream of advice from their loved ones only makes them less and less sure of themselves. "You should try this! Why don't you give her that? You're covering her up too much. . . ." The nanny suggests they consult an allergy specialist. The doctor strongly suspects CMPA and instructs the parents to switch to a brand without cow's milk protein. The digestive problems disappear in a few days, and Mom and Dad are extremely relieved. And so is Sarah.

When baby wheezes . . .
Little Corentin is two months old and has been making strange sounds after finishing his bottle. His parents are worried. Until now, he drank his formula without any problems. Now

he's covered in little bumps that look like hives and he often coughs at night. Recently, he was even hospitalized because he was wheezing "just like someone having an asthma attack," his mother says. She knows what she's talking about. As a child, she would have an asthma attack any time she went near a cat. Corentin's parents take him to the emergency room where the baby is quickly seen by the on-call physician, who understands exactly what is happening. This is an immediate allergic reaction to cow's milk protein that could potentially turn anaphylactic. Thanks to the proper treatment, everything turns out all right. Corentin returns home with formula that does not contain cow's milk protein and an allergy test scheduled for a few weeks later.

Terrible trouble . . .
Young Matheo looks like a little angel. There's just one problem: at around eight months, he develops atopic eczema all over his body. Several other people in his family have allergies, too. He started eating solid foods at the age of six months, but the different formulas he has tried in the past all have given him digestive problems and reflux. Their family doctor suggests they see an allergist, who diagnoses a delayed onset cow's milk protein allergy. They decide to remove cow's milk protein from Matheo's diet and replace it with a product for infants that is rich in casein hydrolysate.

When Matheo is two, he accidentally eats a piece of veal during dinner with his family. The eczema patches on his body return.

When Matheo is three, milk is reintroduced into his diet following a strict protocol. Cooked milk products are added first. He can now eat baked goods containing milk and cheese in small quantities.

Milk and . . . beef?

Little Clara is born in 2014. Her mother breastfeeds her for six months before switching to formula. Then she starts eating solid foods between the ages of six and eight months and—surprise—atopic eczema rears its ugly head.

In 2016, Clara is hospitalized for diarrhea and severe vomiting, leading to a stay in intensive care for dehydration. Milk protein allergy is believed to be the cause of Clara's condition and all dairy products are removed from her diet. In December 2016, after an oral food challenge at the hospital, she is given permission to eat dairy products again.

Her parents also notice that when Clara eats ground beef, she experiences the same kind of vomiting and diarrhea. The symptoms are identical when she eats turkey.

At age three, Clara undergoes another oral food challenge with cow's milk and everything goes smoothly. A milk tolerance protocol is set up, and after two months she is able to consume 150 ml of cow's milk.

Clara's mother is allergic to latex and her father has had eczema since he was a small child. If we look back at the family's interviews with the allergist, we read that Clara had been put on Neocate as part of a dairy elimination diet around the age of one, but that she continued to consume meat, goat's milk, and yogurts made with cow's milk.

Two weeks after the first reintroduction of cow's milk in December 2016 when Clara is allowed to start eating one yogurt a day, the little girl presents with soft stools and severe fatigue. Cow's milk proteins are eliminated once more.

When bottles cause a cough

Chloé is a little bundle of joy. She was born at full term in 2019. For the first three days of her life, she is fed half the time with formula, half the time with breastmilk. This is when the trouble starts: bloating, digestive problems, and an extremely runny nose. Her parents start to get worried because she has started breathing noisily after each bottle.

The parents try two brands of formula without success. Chloé still screams after each bottle. Her father works in the medical field and thinks his daughter's breathing is getting worse. Chloé eventually starts refusing bottles. After consulting an allergist, who suspects an allergy to cow's milk protein, the baby is put on a special formula without cow's milk proteins that is rich in amino acids. In a few days, Chloé is doing much better, sleeping peacefully at night, and gaining weight normally.

Each and every milk . . .

Little Julien lives with his parents in an apartment. The family has two pets: a dog and a cat. Allergies run in the family and his dad is asthmatic. Julien's is quite a story. At six months, he is fed some baby food containing milk. Within minutes he starts coughing and seems to be having trouble breathing. His voice changes and his body breaks out in hives. Horrified, his parents rush him to the hospital. A few weeks later, allergy testing shows that Julien is not only allergic to cow's milk, but to goat's and sheep's milk, too. His doctors start him on an elimination diet and many months go by. Cow's milk is then reintroduced under medical supervision, and Julien's parents also keep an epinephrine auto-injector on them at all times. Goat's and sheep's milk are still off-limits.

Reflux

Flore was born in 2015. Her mother breastfeeds her for three months before switching to formula. After her second bottle, Flore starts vomiting and develops eczema. She cries after every bottle, diarrhea kicks in, and she starts losing weight. Her pediatrician prescribes a rice milk formula made specifically for babies. Flore's digestion still appears to be quite painful, but the eczema disappears. She gains back the weight she lost but her abdominal pain and regurgitation persist until she is one year old. An EGD (esophagogastroduodenoscopy) is performed and reveals gastroesophageal reflux, which is a sign of a non-IgE-mediated allergy to milk. The rice formula is replaced with an amino acid–based milk to reduce the reflux.

More on milk

Milk is understood to be the integral product of the complete and uninterrupted milking of a female dairy animal that is in good health, well-nourished, and not overworked. It should be collected properly and should not contain colostrum. All milk from a female dairy animal other than a cow must include the name of the animal species along with the word "milk." Even a century ago, a clear distinction was made between cow's milk and milk from sheep or goats—and for good reason! Here's a little more information about our infamous allergen.

Whole cow's milk contains 34 g/l of lipids, and semi-skimmed milk contains half that (16 g/l). Skim milk contains less than 0.1 g/l of lipids.

Around thirty allergy-causing proteins have been identified in cow's milk, and they exist in quantities at four times the levels contained in breastmilk.

Carbohydrates with low sugar content like lactose can, over time, lead to lactose intolerance linked to an enzymatic deficiency.

Cow's milk also introduces other elements to the body such as vitamins, hormones, calcium, and residues of antibiotics that the cow has ingested.

The term "dairy product" refers to yogurts, cheeses, creams, butter, and whey, and also casein, which is used in the food and cosmetic industries.

What about plant-based milks?

It is completely misguided to think that the solution when faced with a cow's milk protein allergy is to replace formula with plant-based milks—they are not really milks at all!

A few years ago, in fact, plant-based drinks were evaluated for their nutritional value by the French Agency for Food, Environmental and Occupational Health & Safety (ANSES) following reports of malnutrition in infants under one who were being fed partially or exclusively with these products. These drinks are not made to feed a baby and will cause deficiencies in iron, calcium, and a variety of other vitamins that a baby needs to grow normally. These products simply do not meet the daily nutritional needs of children that age, and for this reason they have no place in the management of a cow's milk protein allergy, no matter how old the child is.

Soy-based products contain high levels of phytoestrogens (isoflavones*) and are strongly discouraged for children under the age of three, pregnant women, and people with a family history of breast cancer. It is also important to keep in mind that there is a possible cross-reactivity between soy and cow's milk.

As ANSES notes, European directive 2006/141/CE (December 22, 2006) stipulates the following: "Infant formula is the only processed foodstuff which wholly satisfies the nutritional requirements of infants during the first months of life until the introduction of appropriate complementary feeding. In order to safeguard the health of such infants it is necessary to ensure that the only products marketed as suitable for such use during the period would be infant formulae."**

---

* These are similar in structure to female estrogen hormones.
** Saisine no. 2011-SA-0261.

Even calcium-enriched almond milk deserves intense scrutiny—as Marie Lossy* pointed out to me, one look at the label reveals that this beverage contains a disappointingly low percentage of almonds. I examined the brand I drink (yes, I'm lactose intolerant) and here's what I found on the label of my liter of almond "milk":

Water, sugar, almond (2.3 percent), sea salt, and carob bean flour as a stabilizer with added emulsifiers. There are other brands that go as high as 7 percent almonds . . . a record! At the end of this book, you'll find Marie Lossy's recipe for homemade plant-based drinks for people who are lactose intolerant and not allergic to tree nuts** (talk to your doctor about how to make sure you're getting enough calcium).

Are hypoallergenic formulas helpful?

Hypoallergenic formula does not help prevent CMPA, and is not useful as a substitution solution. For decades, new mothers have been encouraged to use hypoallergenic (HA) formula made with partially hydrolyzed proteins the moment they leave the hospital, but recent studies have shed new light on whether they actually work to prevent allergies as effectively as the medical establishment has often claimed.

---

* Marie Lossy is the mother of a child with multiple food allergies. See Appendix 1.
** See page 223.

Consider the French Longitudinal Study of Children (ELFE),* which is a wide-ranging child development study that began in 2011. Let's take a moment to say "hurray!" for the funding that is making this long and fruitful endeavor possible. ELFE is the first study of its kind in France and will follow a cohort of eighteen thousand children from birth until the age of twenty.

Participating families were recruited in hospital maternity units throughout France at various periods during the year 2011. Information about the study was presented to randomly selected parents who then answered a questionnaire. As the study progresses, the parents will continue to be interviewed regularly about social, environmental, and medical aspects of their child's life. Since each child's diet is studied closely as part of this project, allergy experts have been able to discover a wealth of new information that has overturned things we had always taken for granted, particularly with regards to the "advantages" of partially hydrolyzed hypoallergenic formulas.

In spite of the fact that medical professionals have been touting their "protective effects" for so many years, thanks to the ELFE study and other publications this idea has fallen out of

---

* The ELFE study is a collaboration between INED (French Institute for Demographic Studies), INSERM (French National Institute of Health and Medical Research), EFS (French National Blood Service), InVS (French Institute for Public Health Surveillance), INSEE (National Institute of Statistics and Economic Studies), the French Ministry of the Ecological Transition, the French Ministry of Solidarity and Health, and CNAF (French National Family Benefits Fund), with the support of the French Ministry of Higher Education, Research and Innovation, CCDSHS (French National Data Committee in Humanities and Social Sciences), and the French Ministry of Culture.

the sky like a lead balloon. The truth is that they do not in any way prevent allergies in children from atopic families, and **using these products at two months may in fact be associated with an increased risk of wheezing at age one and food allergies beginning at age two.** This observation goes against so much of what health professionals have been recommending up until now and additional studies will have to support this observation. A new piece of European legislation plans to require clinical studies on these products before they are allowed to be promoted as having a preventive effect on allergy development.

Needless to say, hypoallergenic formula is also a terrible idea for babies who are allergic to cow's milk protein because it contains partially hydrolyzed forms of these very proteins which—obviously—still pose an allergy risk.

What is a "dangerous bottle"?

When a baby with a family history of allergies is born, parents often wonder things like, "How can we prevent CMPA?" and "What should we feed the baby while we're at the hospital?"

Most studies indicate that supplementing breastmilk with formula during the first three days of life could increase the risk of CMPA in babies with high atopic risk. This is why it is sometimes referred to as a "dangerous bottle."

A better option during the first few days is supplementing with a hydrolysate-based formula or one rich in amino acids, at least while the mother's milk is coming in or for the baby's first month. An article published in late 2019 offers new insight into the prevention of CMPA. Researchers studied two cohorts of newborns with atopic family history—let's take a look at what they discovered:

- For the first three days after birth, the first group of newborns was fed exclusively with breastmilk and, when necessary, a supplement of amino acid–based formula without cow's milk protein.
- For the same length of time, the babies in the second group were breastfed and supplemented with cow's milk–based formula.

There is a striking difference in the way these two groups of children developed over the next two years: children from the first group, who were not given cow's milk for the first three days, developed significantly less CMPA than the second group.

Given this information, new mothers who are breastfeeding should avoid supplementing with cow's milk protein–based products for at least the first three days.

It should also be noted that breastfeeding longer does not prevent the development of CMPA.

Summing it up

If a baby has a family history of allergies and Mom wants to breastfeed and supplement with formula, she should use a hydrolysate- or amino acid–based formula for the first three days after the baby is born.

Regular baby formula can be introduced after this point as long as the child is not allergic to cow's milk protein.

Some numbers

In the United States, CMPA affects 2–3 percent of infants and approximately 0.5 percent of breastfed infants. CMPA risk factors include asthma, eczema, rhinitis or seasonal allergies, and sometimes other food allergies as well.

Several kinds of CMPA

Some people assume that there is only one kind of CMPA, but actually several have been reported. What sets them apart is the timeline of symptoms and the reaction mechanism.

Let's examine each one.

Before we go further, remember that an allergy is an immune system issue and has nothing at all to do with lactose intolerance, which is caused by a deficit of the enzyme lactase.

Immediate IgE-mediated CMPA

If symptoms start within a few minutes or up to two hours after a baby consumes breastmilk containing milk proteins, regular or hypoallergenic formula, or dairy products, you can be fairly certain that you are dealing with an immediate IgE-mediated reaction. Symptoms in this case range from hives to angioedema with swelling of the lips, eyelids, or face. If the throat is affected, there may also be trouble swallowing. In the event of an asthma attack or wheezing, an injection of epinephrine should be administered as quickly as possible as this is a sign of anaphylaxis.

When a baby shows signs of an immediate cow's milk protein allergy, **diagnosis** begins with a detailed interview followed by skin prick tests for cow's milk on the baby's back. Testing can be performed in infants as young as a few weeks old. Blood samples will also be taken and tested for milk allergen-specific IgE antibodies. If necessary, an oral food challenge will sometimes be used to confirm the allergy or to determine how much milk a baby can consume without symptoms. Specialists always aim for as precise a diagnosis as possible in the hopes of avoiding a restrictive diet that may be either inappropriate or ineffective.

Major milk allergens

Casein

Also known as Bos d 8. This protein is thermostable, meaning it is not destroyed by heat, and exists in four forms: alpha s 1, alpha s 2, beta, and kappa. An allergy to this protein may be a sign of persistent CMPA if the level of anti-casein IgE antibodies is above 20 ku/l. In 85 percent of cases, the caseins present in goat's and sheep's milk are similar in structure to the casein in cow's milk, which explains the possible cross-reactivity between these milks.

Beta-lactoglobulin

Bos d 5 is a heat-sensitive protein that accounts for 10 percent of whey proteins. While typically absent from breastmilk, it can appear in the mother's milk if she ingests large amounts of dairy products.

Alpha-lactalbumin

This protein also goes by Bos d 4 and is sensitive to heat.

Albumin

Designated Bos d 6, it is moderately sensitive to heat and is responsible for the cross-reactivity between meat and animal dander.

Summing it up

The proteins we've talked about are found in cow's milk in the following proportions:
- Caseins: 80%
- Whey: 20% (includes 10% beta-lactoglobulin, 5% alpha-lactalbumin, 1% albumin, 3% immunoglobulins, and traces of lactoferrin)

Non-IgE-mediated CMPA

Eczema breakouts, acute or chronic diarrhea accompanied by weight loss, constipation or abdominal pain, gas, reflux, and vomiting are all signs of a non-IgE-mediated allergy mechanism. There is no risk of anaphylaxis unless this allergy happens to be associated with an immediate allergy. If a baby is experiencing major digestive discomfort on a daily basis with chronic eczema breakouts and is failing to gain weight normally, parents should save themselves the countless trips to the pediatrician's office and look into testing for CMPA, which could very likely be the cause.*

Which formulas are safe for a baby with CMPA?

It goes without saying that cow's milk proteins will most likely need to be eliminated from your baby's diet depending on the

---

* Eosinophilic esophagitis and FPIES are explained beginning on page 22.

allergy test results. If so, to meet their child's nutritional needs, parents can choose from a range of what are called "extensively hydrolyzed formulas." These are high in protein but the milk proteins they contain are broken down to such an extent that they are stripped of their allergy-causing potential. Goat's, sheep's, donkey's, and horse's milk should not be used because of the risk of cross-reactivity, and neither should hypoallergenic formula.

Hydrolysate-based formulas for babies with CMPA
Casein hydrolysate options: Enfamil Nutramigen, Enfamil Pregestimil, Similac Alimentum, Similac Expert Care.

Rice-based baby formulas
Enfamil Nutramigen offers rice-based baby forumlas.

These products are entirely unlike the plant-based drinks sold in stores which, as I have already mentioned, should never be used as a substitution drink in children with CMPA.

In severe cases of CMPA, amino acid–based formulas are considered the best option. While they are certainly effective, unfortunately babies do not always take to the flavor. According to one recent study, 17 percent of parents had to go back to the doctor who started them on an amino-acid based formula because their baby refused to drink it.

Amino acid–based formulas
Neocate, Puramino, Nutramigen AA.

If a mother is still breastfeeding, she will need to eliminate milk and dairy products from her diet and supplement her calcium levels with help from her doctor.

In some cases, oral immunotherapy treatment (OIT) can help patients with CMPA build up a tolerance for baked milk products. This treatment must be administered and monitored by an experienced medical team and parents should never attempt this kind of program on their own.

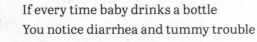

If every time baby drinks a bottle
You notice diarrhea and tummy trouble
Talk to your doctor on the double
Because CMPA could be the missing piece in this puzzle.
Once the culprit cow's milk has been eliminated
It's time to substitute—your baby has been liberated!
There are plenty to choose from, most options are great
And whether it's amino acid or hydrolysate
The greatest comfort is knowing your newborn will gain
    weight.

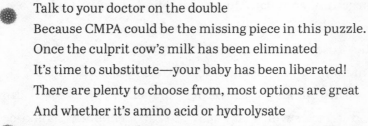

The Essure saga: Was this really a nickel allergy?

When the permanent birth control device Essure was removed from the French market in 2017, many people thought the debate over the explosion of side effects recorded by the French Agency for Food, Environmental and Occupational Health & Safety (ANSES) was over. But even though the problems were initially attributed to a nickel allergy, new studies point to something else. (It's worth noting that in the United States, the FDA had approved Essure in 2002 and that approval was subsequently withdrawn, as well.)

Let's go through the events that took place to understand the tangled web that this affair became.

Essure first appeared on the market in 2002 as a less invasive alternative to tubal ligation. The method seems simple enough: a tiny metal coil is inserted into each fallopian tube and causes scar tissue to build up. After three months, the passage of sperm to the egg is completely blocked.

As the years went by, more and more women with these implants found themselves experiencing violent abdominal pain as well as muscle and/or joint pain a few hours after implantation and even months or years later. Some experienced intense fatigue that was so extreme they had to quit their jobs. Memory problems and hair loss were also reported. The list of symptoms started to grow as more and more women contacted RESIST, a French organization created in 2016 to support Essure victims. Reports continued flooding in and the stories these women shared were chilling. One of those stories belongs to Marielle Klein, the organization's founder. She shared her experience with the French media group Konbini in 2018. Klein received the implant in 2011 and had her first symptoms in 2013. It started with digestive trouble, heart palpitations, and feeling like a "lead blanket" had been placed on top of her. Two years later, she suddenly went deaf from a chronic ear infection and experienced neurological and vision problems as well as muscle spasms. "I was slowly fading away," she says. Her doctors initially dismissed it all as a case of burnout, but she had the strength to fight back and eventually discovered the negative side effects of the device through an American Facebook group called Essure Problems.

Before long, concerns about the side effects reached the ears of the French National Agency for the Safety of Medicines and Health Products (ANSM). In 2015, faced with the growing number of cases, the French Ministry of Solidarity and Health took action and declared that the device could only be implanted by gynecologists or obstetricians who had extensive experience performing operative hysteroscopy. It was not until September 2017 that the device was officially banned from the European market. In the United States it remained in use until 2019, at which point the manufacturer released a terse statement about discontinuing further sales of the product.

The first explanation offered for the negative side effects was a delayed allergic reaction to nickel, one of several metals— including chromium, titanium, tin, iron, silver, platinum, and iridium—contained in the 4-centimeter implants. As a result, for years allergists had women coming to them who were distraught, exhausted, and desperate for help. The medical establishment in France eventually decided that removal of the device was justified if a woman had positive skin tests proving that she was allergic to nickel. But then, thanks to people like Françoise Vanmuysen, a surgeon who was also an Essure victim herself, things started to evolve from a new angle. After having her device removed—a procedure that was accompanied by a hysterectomy with fallopian tube removal—biopsies of her uterine horns were sent to a laboratory for testing. The results provided incontrovertible evidence that this was not an allergy but in fact a problem caused by the release of toxic heavy metals. Researchers began to wonder if the corrosion of the tin in the coil's welding was responsible. A 2020 article in the journal *Dermatitis* refuted once and for all the connection between a nickel allergy and the post-implantation symptoms, and device removal has since been extended to all women with clinical symptoms, even those without positive allergy tests.

On December 22, 2020, a delegation of physicians, Essure victims, and researchers—among them was Dr. Vincent, the medical director of the lab where the mineralogical analysis was performed—announced the results of a study performed on eighteen women who underwent surgical removal of the device. Biopsies and anatomopathological examination had confirmed the presence of tin particles woven into the subjects' uterine tissues, and researchers thought this metal may have subsequently been transformed into a neurotoxin called organotin. There is no doubt that these astonishing new results are an important step toward understanding this phenomenon.

As current RESIST president Émilie Gillier notes, "The majority of women who discover something is wrong with the device want it removed. Very few of them want to keep their implants even if they have not been experiencing severe side effects." Because more and more women are having the device removed and because this procedure is far from risk-free, a detailed surgical protocol has been in place since 2018. To underline how important this protocol is, in September 2020 RESIST addressed a letter to the French Medical Council with information about device removal and the list of reported negative side effects. Gillier is also hopeful that an upcoming French Medical Council bulletin covering the Essure issue will help raise awareness: "We hope that sharing as much information as we can about Essure will alert more women who could benefit from this research. We also want to encourage victims to continue seeking medical care both before and after device removal. And we cannot stress enough how important it is for surgeons to follow the protocol to the letter and schedule an abdominal X-ray before going ahead with the removal procedure—unfortunately not all surgeons do this."

This is not, then, the case of an allergy to nickel, but the body's reaction to toxic metals released by the device's defective tin solders.

In order to better support victims and make sure they receive the best care possible, RESIST has several objectives it hopes to achieve in collaboration with the other entities concerned. The organization has also filed a lawsuit against the manufacturer.

These objectives include:

- Sending a letter to all of the women in France and its overseas territories who currently have the implant informing them of the risks involved with using this device. Unfortunately, for the time being it is not possible to access this kind of information. In fact, even today, women with the implant are still contacting organizations like RESIST desperate to know what's wrong with them but with no knowledge of the risks and research we have discussed here.

• In December 2021, Gillier spoke about the organization's legal proceedings: "Our lawsuit targets the manufacturer directly on the basis of nondisclosure of information to patients and the defectiveness of the medical device. What we hope is that a judge will approve the lawsuit, which would allow all of the victims to attach their complaints to ours. . . . We want victims to know that there are always volunteers available to answer their questions and that the women in our organization will never stop working to keep the chain of solidarity, support, and outreach going."

To the women who are victims of this injustice,
    this is for you.
Even if you have only minor symptoms, here's the best
    course of action to pursue:
Contact a support group as soon as you can
And in this tight-knit community
May you find comfort and solidarity!

Amazing allergy research from Japan

Most scientists have their noses buried in their work and their heads in the clouds. But luckily for us, some of them find the time to research things that are truly amusing and truly fascinating. This is exactly what Japanese physician Dr. Hajime Kimata has been doing for years.

Dr. Kimata's work explores the interaction between humor and the evolution of disease, specifically allergies, and is inspired by the writings of American journalist Norman Cousins. Cousins, after being diagnosed with ankylosing spondylitis, wrote a book called *Anatomy of an Illness as Perceived by the Patient* describing how he battled this inflammatory disease using the rather unconventional method of checking into a hotel, taking vitamin C, and watching Marx Brothers comedies. Believe it or not, this "laugh therapy" had a positive impact on the progression of his illness.

Healing with a kiss

But let's get back to Dr. Kimata's eclectic work. In 2003, he conducted a study to find out if kissing could alleviate or prevent the appearance of allergy symptoms. Over the course of the experiment, Kimata studied three groups of thirty people. One cohort was made up of people with allergic rhinitis. The second consisted of patients suffering from atopic eczema. Members of both groups were allergic to dust mites and cedar pollen. The last group was a control group without allergies. All of the people in the study were of Japanese origin and kissing on a regular basis was not customary for any of them. Behind closed doors, each of the study participants enjoyed thirty minutes of kissing his or her partner while listening to romantic songs like Celine Dion's "My Heart Will Go On." After the kissing, the subjects' allergen skin tests were less reactive than they had been before the study. The study concluded that love and passionate kisses were capable of reducing the intensity of an allergic response. This is certainly something worth keeping in mind, except of course in the case of a food allergy when a kiss could prove deadly.*

Note

The study I just mentioned was honored at the 25th Annual Ig Nobel Prize ceremony in Cambridge, Massachusetts. This annual gathering is organized by the magazine **Annals of Improbable Research** (AIR). The Ig Nobel Prize in medicine bestowed upon Dr. Kimata was shared with three Slovakian scientists who were recognized for their work on the persistence of male DNA in the female oral cavity after intense kissing. What a lineup!

Therapeutic laughter

Kimata was off to such a good start that he just kept going. His bibliography is peppered with other treasures like the study he conducted in 2004 to determine whether laughter could affect allergic skin responses in patients with atopic eczema. Participants were asked to watch a funny *Mr. Bean* video or a weather report. Allergic skin responses were reduced after participants had watched the funny film. Since there was nothing amusing about the weather report, there was no change in the

---

*   See page 129.

allergic response after participants viewed it. When they were given a stressful task—in this case composing text messages on a mobile phone—the participants experienced an increased allergic response. Interestingly, however, watching the *Mr. Bean* video before the texting counteracted its negative effects. The study concluded that patients with atopic eczema should compose their text messages while watching comedies.

In 2008, the same author set out to discover what impact comedy might have on erectile dysfunction in men with atopic eczema. Once again, it proved to have a positive effect. The research team started from the premise that an eczema flare-up negatively impacted the participants' powers of seduction, sexual performance, and testosterone secretion. The study was aiming to find a solution to these "defects." Thirty-six men with atopic eczema and their healthy partners were split into two groups. One watched comedies for three days in a row: *Mr. Bean, Modern Times*, and *There's Something About Mary*. Two weeks later, the same group watched long, informational films without a single trace of humor. The other group did the reverse. To prevent the results from being skewed, no vibrators or sex toys could be used during the study. Blood samples were taken to measure testosterone and estradiol levels and the results were remarkable: watching comedies significantly increased testosterone production for a period of four days. This very encouraging result improved the men's erectile function, sexual desire, and orgasm while allowing them to "forget their eczema."

Music therapy

In his quest for allergy knowledge, the insatiable Dr. Kimata has even examined the relationship between classical music and latex allergy symptoms! Did you know that listening to Mozart reduces the skin's allergic response to latex as well as the level of latex-specific IgE antibodies in the blood? In case you were wondering, the same cannot be said for Beethoven's symphonies!

Reading through this plethora of scientific publications on such a variety of topics makes me rather jealous. I have to admit that I would have loved to be part of his team!

Do you have allergies?
Do you wish managing them was more of a breeze?
Well don't leave it to chance
And listen to Mozart next time you want to dance.
Then French kiss someone
From dusk until dawn
And watch comedies for the rest of your life!

CHAPTER 4

Allergies and COVID-19

In this chapter, we're going to set aside the pangolins, bats, and other theories about the origin of COVID-19 and instead focus on how this difficult period has affected allergy management.

Inhaled corticosteroids for the treatment of asthma

Since March 2020, our lives been turned upside down by a little virus that has proved to be a nasty piece of work. It has viciously attacked our elderly loved ones and affected people from every sector of the population. Very early on, the question of whether or not allergy and asthma treatments containing corticosteroids could exacerbate COVID-19 symptoms became an important issue. Keep in mind that between January and October, a mob of dancing pollen grains goes soaring through the air and causing trouble for allergy sufferers. Treatment of symptoms involves the daily use of antihistamines and inhaled corticosteroids. When those symptoms evolve to include a nose that is completely congested and endless sneezing that the usual treatment can no longer handle, additional corticosteroids are taken orally for a few days. In the case of asthma, treatment typically includes inhaled corticosteroids that are taken alone or in conjunction with long-acting bronchodilators that are prescribed for long-term use. At the beginning of the pandemic, warnings about NSAID use making COVID-19 symptoms worse made the rounds in the media. Naturally, people started to get worried and seeds of doubt suddenly sprouted in their minds. Some decided to abruptly stop their inhaled corticosteroid treatments, which caused problems with their asthma. Physicians realized that they needed to take action quickly and announced that there was absolutely no reason for people currently using inhaled corticosteroids to stop taking them under any circumstances since the amount of time these medications spend in the bloodstream is nearly nonexistent under usual doses. The Asthma and Allergy Working Group of the French Society of Respiratory Diseases (SPLF) also published a statement confirming that background asthma treatments should be maintained at an effective dose during the COVID-19 period.

There has also been concern about asthma being a risk factor for severe forms of COVID-19, which is known to attack the respiratory system, but recent studies do not seem to suggest this, especially if the asthma is allergy-related and well-controlled. Severe forms of asthma, however, may pose a greater risk of respiratory distress in the event of a COVID-19 infection. If symptoms like muscle pains, headache, diarrhea, hyperthermia, and sudden loss of smell are accompanied by exacerbated asthma symptoms, this could be a sign of a COVID-19 infection.

Hay fever

The 2020 pollen season—the summer in particular—was an aggressive one in many parts of the world for a number of reasons. First, any location with mild weather allowed pollen to spread in greater numbers than usual, and second, in countries that were locked down for the first time, parks, roadsides, and open areas could not be cleared, which meant there were more weed and grass plants releasing pollen. But knowing this information about a previous year is not necessarily useful for people with allergies because they have to be prepared for the worst every year. Spring kicks off with the spread of grass seed pollen, which causes what is usually called "hay fever" (cases were less severe than usual in 2021), and ends with a flourish of weed pollen. Allergy sufferers should also keep in mind that exposure to air pollution, particularly fine particles and diesel fuel, intensifies pollen's allergenic potential. This is because air pollutants damage the pollen grains, allowing more pollen to be released into the environment. This interaction also alters the pollen's composition and actually has the power to make it more allergenic than pollen in an unpolluted area. Allergenic pollen that is anemophilous (carried by the wind) can increase allergy symptoms in people whose airways are already fragile as a result of preexisting asthma or irritation from volatile organic compounds polluting the air around them.

Another issue for allergic individuals is the confirmed fact that the length of allergy season has been increasing every year. Global warming is not unrelated to this phenomenon. Thanks to increasing temperatures, pollens like those from the cypress tree can be transported over larger geographical areas by the wind, which means more and more people are then affected by this allergy.

For all of these reasons, anyone with allergies should talk to his or her allergist and set up a treatment plan that can begin before allergy season starts.

COVID-19 certainly created a topsy-turvy time, but I'd like to remind everyone that allergen desensitization therapies can be continued or started as long as there is no risk of infection and as long as the patient does not belong to one of the following groups: children under the age of five, people with unstable asthma or neoplasia, people taking beta blockers, or women in early pregnancy. Note that a desensitization therapy that was started well before pregnancy can be continued during it, but this kind of treatment should not be started during the pregnancy. If you are a patient receiving sublingual specific immunotherapy and you develop a fever, treatment should be stopped and you should contact your allergist to find out what to do. A PCR test and self-isolation while you wait for the results is the best idea.

Protective masks

There has been a significant amount of back-and-forth about how helpful masks really are, but no one can deny that they were once a part of our daily lives and have become one tool people use to protect themselves. This only works, of course, if the mask is worn properly. If someone is wearing a surgical mask, for example, the metal clip at the top should be pinched over the nose and the blue or pink side should be facing out. Wearing a mask under the nose or on the chin defeats its purpose entirely, and complaining that it's always sliding down is just a bad excuse. Despite what certain people may say, there is no risk of oxygen desaturation when it is worn for several hours.

I think most people can agree that wearing a mask is far from practical, especially for those of us who have to go around with perpetually fogged-up glasses. During the pandemic, many of us became used to putting up with what has come to be known as "maskne" around the lips and on the cheeks and chin. This phenomenon is often the result of the mask rubbing and irritating skin on the face that is already aggravated by heat and moisture inside the mask. To combat this, apply a soap and fragrance-free facial cleanser locally and always follow with a fragrance-free moisturizer.

Some people like to put their own spin on these infamous masks and choose the color and shape that suits them. Allergic reactions to masks are very rare and should not be confused with irritations, but a person who is allergic to PPD (the same allergen that is present in hair dye) is likely to have a reaction if his or her mask has been dyed black. Other mask wearers, as a November 2021 article in the *Revue française d'allergologie* reports, may develop a contact allergy to the rubber accelerators in the mask's elastic straps.

Just about any doctor will strongly recommend wearing sunscreen in the summer. But does this advice still apply if we're wearing a surgical mask half of the time? Yes, but you need to be careful about which creams you use and where you apply them. A recent study has confirmed that masks do protect from the sun's UVA and UVB rays, so try to avoid using a chemical sunscreen anywhere except your forehead and temples. Any chemicals in the creams and tinted moisturizers you use on a daily basis will penetrate the skin inside your mask more than before. This is because rubbing and prolonged face mask use makes skin more permeable and sensitive to products that are applied to it. Unfortunately, this is also the ideal trigger for a case of contact eczema caused by the preservatives in cosmetics and perfumes.

Hand sanitizers

Early in the pandemic, stores were constantly running out of alcohol-based hand sanitizers, and now using it has become something we do every day—just like washing our hands. Unfortunately, using it multiple times throughout the day as advised does alter the hydrolipidic film that protects our skin. This is causing all kinds of skin issues to crop up, whether as a result of allergies or simply irritation. It goes without saying that people with eczema or other skin diseases may see these protective measures as a punishment. But, as the French Society of Dermatology has noted, it is in fact handwashing and not the use of hand sanitizers that causes skin abrasions. The skin allergy specialists in this academic society wrote a guide on this topic and suggest watching for the early signs of an irritation (a burning sensation, not itching). If this happens, pamper your skin by washing with fragrance-free soaps or syndets (synthetic detergents) and warm water before carefully drying your hands. You can moisturize with a fragrance-free emollient cream, but don't apply it right after applying hand sanitizer or you risk diminishing the effectiveness of both products. If you apply moisturizer before bed, you can sleep while your hands soak up the hydration!

When choosing a hand sanitizer, it's a good idea to look for one that won't titillate your nostrils with the strong scent of essential oils; these could trigger allergy symptoms or irritations in people with asthma and allergies.

You may be thinking about protective gloves as a potential solution, but if a person already has eczema, he or she is out of luck because these gloves increase local hyperhidrosis (sweating) and therefore increase skin maceration. If you don't have eczema and are someone who wears protective gloves on a regular basis, don't be afraid to apply hand lotion frequently.

Most importantly, if you are taking an immunosuppressant like cyclosporine or methotrexate for your eczema and have questions about your risk of contracting COVID-19, contact your dermatologist. He or she will tell you whether to continue or modify your treatment.

Vaccination and anaphylaxis

In 2020, SARS-CoV-2 became our mortal enemy and sent scientists around the world on a race to develop vaccines to battle it. The US vaccination campaign started in 2021 and continued to pick up speed. Early in the campaign, the specter of vaccine anaphylaxis peeked its head out. The first two cases of this were reported in Great Britain. The individuals had received the Pfizer vaccine and were known to have severe allergies.

Without getting alarmed, you should be aware that this rare reaction was reported in other countries as well. Do not give into panic by rushing to see an allergist. Remember that the incidence of allergies to these new vaccines remains comparable to that of other vaccines. Currently, the risk of allergy to the Pfizer vaccine is estimated to be 11.1 cases for every 1 million injections.

The guilty parties can be placed in a variety of categories, but polyethylene glycol (PEG) was the first one mentioned in the rare cases of anaphylaxis that were observed after injection with the Pfizer-BioNTech vaccine. PEG can be found in cosmetics (creams, hair conditioners) and medical products (lubricating gels, suppositories). Other forms of PEG, specifically PEG 3350 and PEG 4000, are present in osmotic laxatives. These last two are the ones to watch out for if you have allergies. Here's what you need to know:

- You may have already absorbed or applied PEG 3350 and/or PEG 4000 without realizing it and had no reaction. You do not need to worry and this is not a reason to avoid getting a vaccine.
- If, on the other hand, you have a history of allergies to PEG 3350 and/or PEG 4000 and have had reactions in

the past to laxatives and medications used to prepare for a colonoscopy, contact your allergist. PEGs with high molecular weight seem to be the ones causing problems.

The rest of the COVID-19 vaccines contain a list of other potential suspects. One of them, polysorbate 80 (AstraZeneca), is commonly found in injectable medications that are already on the market and in many other vaccines. It is also present in food as polysorbate 80 (E 433). This substance has been known to cause anaphylaxis in very rare cases. During the first injections of the Moderna vaccine in the United States in late 2020, ten cases of anaphylaxis within less than fifteen minutes were observed. This amounts to 2.5 observed cases for every 1 million doses administered.

In April 2021, fifty-eight allergic reactions were reported to the French National Agency for the Safety of Medicines and Health Products (ANSM) out of the 10 million doses of Comirnaty Pfizer/BioNTech vaccine that were administered.

Tromethamine, a common ingredient in several contrast agents, is another potential troublemaker. Luckily, thanks to quick action, there have been no cases of death linked to this allergy. Anyone with a known allergy to these products should contact their allergist. Skin tests can confirm whether or not you should get vaccinated.

In a press release at the beginning of the vaccine campaign, Professor Frédéric de Blay, president of the French Allergy

Federation (FFAL)*, reminded the public that "30 percent of people in France have allergies and these individuals do not need to consult an allergist before vaccination even if they have severe allergies. Only patients with certain medical history should do so. This history may include severe reactions to an injectable medication, another vaccine, or to an unidentified medication. This information will allow health care professionals to make sure there is nothing preventing these individuals from receiving a vaccine."

This means that people who are allergic to airborne allergens like dust mites, animal dander, pollen, mold, and cockroaches as well as those with food allergies should feel comfortable getting vaccinated without consulting their allergist first.

Health care teams have prepared for all possible scenarios and will monitor the vaccinated individual for fifteen to thirty minutes with injectable epinephrine close at hand in the event of an anaphylactic reaction.

Local reactions like redness and swelling—typically observed in the days just after vaccination—occur with 84 percent of Moderna injections. However, an article in *The New England Journal of Medicine* pointed out that this mRNA vaccine can

---

* The French Allergy Federation (FFAL) includes:
  • The French Allergy Society (SFA)
  • The French Syndicate of Allergists (SYFAL)
  • The French National Association for Continuing Education in Allergology (ANAFORCAL)
  • The French College of Allergology Teachers (CEA)
  • The organizations Asthma and Allergies (A&A) and the French Association for the Prevention of Allergies (AFPRAL)

also produce delayed reactions at eight days post-injection. The reactions mentioned in the article included skin eruptions at least four inches (ten cm) wide accompanied by general symptoms (fever, etc.) that lessened within six days with treatment of these symptoms. The authors did not consider these late-onset reactions a reason not to receive a second injection. Remember, again, that these reactions are the exception and are in no way an argument against vaccination!

As I am sure you noticed, COVID-19 vaccine protocols have evolved and now call for three doses. In France, contraindications to the mRNA vaccines have also expanded to include the following (according to the SFA and FFAL):

- Individuals with documented history of an allergy (proven by allergy tests) to one of the vaccine components (PEG in particular), or who are at risk for cross-reactivity with polysorbate 80.
- Individuals with a history of anaphylaxis affecting at least two organs following the first injection of an mRNA vaccine.

In the event of an anaphylactic reaction, emergency epinephrine will be administered and the patient will be monitored for at least seven hours. Serum tryptase levels will be measured between thirty minutes and two hours after the reaction and tested again twenty-four hours later.

All other allergy history: normal vaccination procedure with fifteen to thirty minutes of post-injection monitoring.

Note: a previous allergic reaction to food or bee stings, no matter how severe, is not a contraindication to vaccination.

A few studies claim to have achieved successful desensitization to the Moderna and Comirnaty vaccines in patients with suspected or confirmed allergic reactions to COVID-19 vaccines. The researchers followed desensitization protocols that have been used for other vaccines and adapted them as needed. This kind of treatment remains rare for the moment and new studies will have to be conducted to refine this specialized protocol.

Post-COVID syndrome and your skin

For some, a COVID-19 infection may be asymptomatic. For others, the symptoms are quite severe and may involve a stay in intensive care for acute respiratory distress. Typically, depending on contact tracing and variants, the US Centers for Disease Control and Prevention recommends five days of isolation followed by five days wearing a mask. After that, everything should be feeling back to normal. Unfortunately, this doesn't always happen. Over time, health care professionals have started observing persistent and at times debilitating symptoms that are lasting for over four weeks after the initial infection. This is what is known as "post-COVID syndrome" or "long COVID."

According to a study that appeared in *The Lancet* in early January 2021, 66–87 percent of infected patients still showed symptoms two months after a positive PCR test. Since many of these prolonged symptoms are skin-related, an international registry of COVID-19 skin manifestations was created to better understand the relationship between the virus and dermatological symptoms. This registry contains reports of hives (usually lasting four to twenty-eight days), papulosquamous eruptions (lasting twenty to seventy days), and chilblains (lasting less than two weeks). This is the information that we have so far, but it could evolve as the pandemic moves further behind us. These skin problems may be accompanied by other symptoms like intense fatigue, digestive trouble, loss of smell (anosmia) and taste (ageusia), neurological and/or heart problems, and difficulty breathing.

Another group of researchers trying to shine a light on the mystery of long COVID is the team behind the COCOLATE study coordinated by Tourcoing Medical Center. This study collects data on patients who did not spend time in intensive care but who are still experiencing at least one symptom two months after they contracted the virus. This project has extended to thirty medical centers around France and hopes to recruit one thousand patients.

In March 2020, Santé publique France, the country's national public health agency, launched a survey as part of a study called CoviPrev tracing the impact of COVID-19 on French people's behavior and mental health during and after lockdown. The results are updated regularly and available to view on their website.

An international survey about allergy management during the pandemic was taken to assess the connection between allergies and COVID-19 risk. Six hundred and thirty-five participants from seventy-eight countries responded to the twenty-four survey questions and the results—which were released in February 2021, before the appearance of new variants—indicate that people with allergies and hypersensitivities do not have a higher risk of contracting COVID-19. There is also no increased risk of infection linked to current allergy and asthma treatments, including biologics like omalizumab, mepolizumab, and dupilumab.

A warning about pholcodine and COVID-19

In an April 2020 press briefing, the French National Agency for the Safety of Medicines and Health Products (ANSM) warned the public against self-medicating with cough medicines containing pholcodine during the COVID-19 period because of the problems they could potentially cause for a patient who needed to be intubated or undergo other interventions in intensive care. Why the concern? Let me explain how all of this relates to allergies.

Pholcodine has been used since the 1950s in cough syrups for children and adults, but today's doctors have it in their crosshairs and are holding it responsible for generating cross-reactivity with neuromuscular blocking agents (muscle relaxants). This cross-reactivity, they believe, could explain why muscle relaxants are the number one drug-related cause of perioperative anaphylaxis. **Note that Pholcodine is not prescribed for use in the United States or Canada.**

For a long time one question has gone unanswered: how can a patient have an anaphylactic response to muscle relaxants with only one exposure? In fact, this allergic reaction is caused by the presence of a quaternary ammonium group in the muscle relaxant's chemical structure. These quaternary ammonium groups also happen to be present in many everyday products (cleaning products, cosmetics, hair dye PPD) and in cough syrups like pholcodine.

Researchers initially hypothesized that patients who had these severe reactions had been previously sensitized via one of these common household products, and epidemiological studies revealed that more females than males were experiencing anaphylaxis after exposure to muscle relaxants. The surge in these cases led Scandinavian scientists to investigate the problem. Pholcodine, they found, was able to increase levels of total IgE antibodies as well as specific IgE antibodies against quaternary ammonium. Pholcodine-based products have, as a result, been banned since 1998 in Sweden and since 2007 in Norway. These countries have seen a significant drop in anaphylaxis related to muscle relaxants.

Cough syrups containing pholcodine*:
    Biocalyptol
    Broncalène
    Clarix
    Diémétane
    Flucalyptol
    Hexapneumine
    Poléry
*Not prescribed for use within the United States or Canada.

Products containing quaternary ammonium:
    Promethazine
    Neostigmine
    Chlorpromazine
    Morphine
    Pholcodine
    PPD in hair dye
    Cosmetics
    Cleaning products

You may be wondering how to find out what ingredients are in your cleaning products. In the US, hazardous cleaning products are marked with a warning symbol and an indication of their possible impact on the environment. The labels on these products will also include a description of their potential dangers and information about proper usage of the product.

Unfortunately, these regulations are not always respected, but a new, clearer label for cleaning products should be released soon. The French Minister of the Ecological Transition, Barbara Pompili, has also proposed a new label that would feature a "Toxi-Score" for all household products.

CHAPTER 5

Allergies, Intimacy, and Sex

In this chapter I will focus on the curious connections between sex and allergy risks. This subject is not often discussed and may sound laughable, but it is something everyone should know about because the clinical symptoms can be severe—ranging from hives to anaphylaxis. Health issues related to our sex lives are very often underdiagnosed because patients sometimes find it difficult to speak openly about their sexual practices and hygiene habits.

And no, we will not be studying the positions of the Kama Sutra.

A kiss, whether it be a peck on the cheek or something more passionate, can be deadly for someone with a food allergy. A much-hoped-for sexual encounter transforms into a catastrophe for someone allergic to semen. And if a condom is used, the parties involved may have to worry about triggering a latex allergy.

I believe that this small selection of cases can be useful to everyone, including health care professionals and sexologists. . . .

Uninvited guests

When allergies show up to a party uninvited, the feverish embrace that two people have been waiting for may turn out to be a test of courage. Here is why.

First of all, making love isn't always a walk in the park. Every man and woman wants to give it their best effort, there is very much a sense of performance involved, and people tend to really put their hearts into it. But sometimes the machine gets stuck and all of a sudden we're looking at possible blood pressure problems, swelling, hives, trouble breathing, anaphylaxis, and even a loss of consciousness. Why? The culprit is an allergy called **food-dependent exercise-induced anaphylaxis (FDEIA)** that occurs when a person ingests a food allergen they are already sensitized to (wheat, shellfish, soy, fruit . . .) and engages in physical effort within the following four hours. It is truly unique because there is no allergic reaction at all if there is no accompanying physical effort (playing sports, dancing, biking, swimming, skiing, etc.) after the person eats the problem food. FDEIA symptoms are often exacerbated by external factors such as drinking, the use of NSAIDs, menstruation, and cold or hot temperatures. Obviously, if something like this happens to you, consult an allergist and keep an epinephrine auto-injector with you just in case. When the allergen is identified, you will have to avoid any physical effort for at least four to six hours after consuming it.

At other times, having sex can sometimes feel like a long-distance race. The runners both need a healthy set of lungs and a heart that is up to the task! When asthma intrudes on this intimate moment, it's no fun at all. You may start wheezing and suddenly find it hard to catch your breath and, naturally, all of this affects sexual performance. If you have asthma and start experiencing these symptoms, it's important that you react quickly and use your inhaler (which should always be nearby!). Your current treatment may not be enough to prevent your symptoms, so consult your doctor to make sure it is up to date. If you have exercise-induced asthma, talk to your doctor and he or she will prescribe an inhaler to use fifteen minutes before having sex.

For people with food allergies, regrettably, kissing can cause allergen sensitization or trigger potentially deadly allergic reactions via **indirect proxy contact** with the allergen. If this sounds improbable to you, then perhaps you have never heard about any of the tragic cases of teenagers losing their lives after a French kiss became a kiss of death—all because their partner had recently eaten a food they were allergic to! Remember this when you invite people with allergies to your home. Is your boyfriend allergic to peanuts or any other foods? Did you eat any before having him over? Wash your hands and mouth before saying hello. The best option, of course, is to avoid consuming any of the culprit food on the day you see each other. Even a kiss on the cheek could be a problem and cause hives, swelling, or even anaphylaxis. And watch out for those little "extras" like edible chocolate body paint that people sometimes use to spice up fore-play. If someone has a milk allergy, using it is probably not the greatest idea of the century. You should be equally cautious with fruit-flavored massage oils and read the list of ingredients before using one.

Public health campaigns have been telling people to use condoms since the 1980s. They protect from all kinds of sexually transmitted diseases (STD) and unwanted pregnancy. But just because you're having protected sex doesn't mean you won't encounter complications like a ripped condom or a **latex allergy**, which happens to be the most common sex-related allergy. Symptoms may include swelling of the vulva or penis, local or generalized hives, and even an asthma attack signaling anaphylaxis as soon as sex begins. Contraceptive methods will most likely have to be adjusted after allergy testing confirms a latex allergy. Obviously, choosing a condom that does not contain latex is the best idea, and today there are many more options than there used to be. Here are a few solutions available for people with allergies:*

- Max Tolérance and Real Feeling, Protex Original 0.02 (note: the Protex Classic contains latex), Manix Skyn, Manix Suprême, Durex Nude.
- Trojan Naturalamb is a condom made from lamb intestine.

- Female condoms (Femindom) are not as glamorous but they are just as effective and should not be passed over. These can be used by people with allergies.
- For people who practice cunnilingus, a dental dam made from polyurethane is one solution. Some brands are made with latex, so check the ingredients and the expiration date before each use.

  Note that some of these brands may not be available in the United States or Canada.

Medical equipment and everyday objects that may contain latex

Certain glues on self-sticking envelopes, balloons, blood pressure cuffs, support stockings, elastic bandages, heating pads, condoms, diaphragms, elastics, sponges, cleaning gloves, surgical gloves, rubber toys, diving equipment (mask, goggles, swimming cap), finger cots, shower curtains, bathmats, bottle nipples and pacifiers, syringe pistons, and probes. Latex is also used in the film industry in synthetic skin for special effects and costumes.

People with latex allergies may be able to breathe easy during unprotected sex, but for women with dog allergies, the moment of ejaculation is not without risk. Some of them will experience an **allergic reaction to their partner's semen** in the thirty minutes following sex. What is the connection between a dog dander allergy and this reaction? In fact, the problem is caused by a cross-reactivity between two allergens, one of which is present in humans and the other in dogs. Human prostate-specific antigen (PSA) is very similar in structure (55–60 percent) to an allergenic protein in dogs called Can f 5 or prostatic kallikrein. This is usually found in the pooch's dander and urine.

The first real documented case of this kind of reaction to semen was recorded by the French scientist Bernard Halpern in 1967. Since then, just over eighty cases have been reported around the globe.

Thirty to 40 percent of women with a semen allergy will begin experiencing symptoms after they have sex for the first time. Whatever part of the body comes into contact with the sperm typically starts burning and itching, which can at first lead to an incorrect diagnosis of vulvovaginitis. The following more serious symptoms may also develop after sex: hives all over the body, local swelling, and early signs of anaphylaxis like asthma attacks, nausea, vomiting, and diarrhea. Women are most susceptible to these reactions between the ages of twenty and thirty.

Diagnosis is based on three criteria:

- Length of time after ejaculation before symptoms appeared.
- Disappearance of symptoms when a condom is used.
- Positive skin test using the sexual partner's semen which is centrifuged for thirty minutes at 39°F (4°C) to separate the sperm from the semen. Sperm is then filtered through a 0.2 μm membrane. The spermatozoa

are not considered to be the cause of the allergic
reaction.
• Blood test results usually reveal the presence of human
semen-specific and Can f 5-specific IgE antibodies.

In April 2019, Japanese researchers published the case of a thir-
ty-seven-year-old woman who had an anaphylactic reaction
thirty minutes after unprotected sex with her husband. She was
found to be sensitized to dog dander and was already aware of
her atopic eczema, but she had never had this kind of problem
until a dog started spending time at her workplace. Whenever
she gave it a pat, her hands would get red and swell, signaling
that she was in fact allergic to the animal.

Ever since the discovery of the dog/semen allergy phenomenon, many scientists have investigated the subject to offer couples
more practical solutions.

If a couple is not trying to conceive, the allergic partner
is encouraged to take an antihistamine thirty minutes before
having sex to avoid very mild reactions to semen. For total
protection from symptoms, however, condoms are also imper-
ative. Abstinence helps, for obvious reasons, but pulling out
before ejaculation produces mixed results.

Progress continues to be made and researchers recently have
had promising results with treatment using a monoclonal antibody called omalizumab.* Here's a quick summary of the case:
After sex during her second pregnancy, the patient, a mother

---

* Anti-IgE antibody typically used to treat asthma and chronic hives.

of two, was hospitalized for anaphylaxis caused by an allergy to semen. She had experienced mild itching before but had not paid any attention to it. After administering epinephrine, the medical team decided to treat her with omalizumab. A year later, the treatment continues to be a success. She no longer uses condoms and has returned to her normal sex life without reacting to her husband's semen.

For couples who are trying to conceive a child, a variety of solutions have been proposed by different medical teams over the past fifteen years. In 1999, one team helped a twenty-nine-year-old woman allergic to semen become a mother on her sixth attempt at artificial insemination using her husband's washed sperm. Unfortunately, 10–20 percent of the time this insemination technique is followed by episodes of anaphylaxis. Other reproductive methods were examined, and in 2006, a woman obtained a full-term pregnancy after the fourth round of in vitro fertilization (IVF) with her husband's sperm. IVF is considered a better option than artificial insemination because it is more effective in preventing these kinds of allergic reactions.

At the fourteenth Francophone Congress of Allergology (CFA) in 2019, a team from Grenoble Alpes University Hospital presented the case of a twenty-five-year-old woman who was allergic to semen and had been married for eight years. She was initially instructed to use a condom. Two years later, she and her husband decided they wanted to have children. After six failed artificial inseminations, the doctors decided to look at intravaginal immunotherapy, which is an effective alternative to assisted reproductive technology. The protocol was based on one used in Angers*, and thanks to this treatment, the woman was able to get pregnant and avoid IVF.

Before assuming the diagnosis is an allergy to semen, it is of course essential to eliminate any other possible causes like yeast infections or STDs.

This cross-reactivity should not be confused with the "burning semen syndrome" described in the early 1990s. To understand the latter, we have to go back to the time of the Gulf War. When they got back home, some veterans noticed burning and swelling of the penis after exposure to their own sperm. After unprotected sex, some of their female partners also suffered symptoms mimicking an allergy. Out of 700,000 soldiers, only 211 mentioned having this problem. The researcher who examined this problem believed that these soldiers had been exposed to chemicals that modified the makeup of their sperm.

Another puzzling sex-related pathology is post-orgasmic illness syndrome (POIS). It is very rare and affects men a few seconds after orgasm and can last up to seven days. Symptoms vary from one individual to another but they can be so severe that some men abstain from sex completely. POIS can show itself in the form of anxiety, flu-like symptoms (fever, sore throat, migraine, shivering, diffuse pain, and intense fatigue), or memory loss after each orgasm. As to its mechanism, there are several theories, but some researchers believe it could be

_____

* Dr. Martine Drouet.

connected to an allergy. For now, though, this phenomenon remains somewhat inexplicable.

Could things possibly get any worse? In a word, yes. Did you know that food allergens could be transmitted during sex and trigger a reaction? The unfortunate events experienced by a woman allergic to Brazil nuts is the perfect illustration of this. After eating a few of these tree nuts, her boyfriend, who knew about her allergy, carefully washed his mouth and brushed his teeth. Later that day when the couple was having unprotected sex, the woman immediately felt burning and swelling around her vulva. Several clues led one allergy specialist to investigate further. The Brazil nut allergen, it turns out, had not been destroyed during digestion and was present in her boyfriend's sperm.

Choosing the right place for the big event

It's a beautiful warm day and two enraptured bodies are lying intertwined and naked in the cool grass. But the next day, this moment of unforgettable ecstasy becomes a nightmare. One lover's skin is itchy, swollen, and covered in blisters. What happened? A textbook case of **meadow dermatitis**, a kind of phytophotodermatitis. For some people, the combination of sun, sweat, and contact with grass has an explosive effect on skin resulting in debilitating skin reactions that leave behind a rather bitter memory of the events that caused them. So if you're thinking of taking a romp with your partner somewhere outdoors, bring a blanket to protect yourself from this unpleasantness. If you or the other person have severe symptoms, head to a doctor to get a prescription for a cortisone cream that can be applied locally.

Even if your plans are indoors, by the way, asking your future sex partner about their allergies can help prevent the long-awaited evening from being spoiled. Imagine if you have a cute little cat who spends its days purring on the couch or lounging in your bed. And then your date arrives. Perhaps she has never mentioned to you that she is highly allergic to cats. The evening becomes a concert of sneezing and her nose is running like a fountain. With red and watery eyes, she looks at you and says that she can't stay or she'll have an asthma attack. Even if you put your kitty outside or in another room for the hours before your hot date, it won't help—cat allergens can linger in the air for at least six months!

Or maybe the problem is that you're not the king or queen of cleaning. Your mattress might be a little old. You may prefer feather pillows. If these things are true and if the person who has won your heart is allergic to dust mites, rhinitis could very well ruin your evening. The same is true if you bring your significant other to your vacation home for the weekend—if the house is unoccupied for most of the year, that means dust mites have had plenty of time to frolic in the bedding.

If your ladylove suggests something naughty while you're reading your morning paper, be aware that newspaper ink can cause contact allergies. Caressing the vulva, for instance, could deposit sensitizing substances in the ink (rosin, varnish, additives, pigments, or colorants) and cause swelling in the pubic area. The moral of the story is to always wash your hands! Or to not read the newspaper before foreplay.

Increasing pleasure

Stimulating the libido is a tempting idea, but sometimes it doesn't always work out as planned.

Ginger, or *Zingiber officinale,* is venerated for its aphrodisiac qualities and it does appear to boost libido, but be warned: it is also the culprit behind rare cases of immediate food allergy reactions, the first of which was mentioned in 1985. Allergies to spices, of which ginger is one, make up 2 percent of all food allergies. People affected by this particular phenomenon are usually young adults, typically female, and often allergic to mugwort or birch pollen.

Like cardamom and turmeric, ginger is a tropical plant in the Zingiberaceae family. According to the few existing articles on the topic, symptoms just after ingestion can range from hives and swelling to asthma attacks and anaphylaxis. An article in the *Revue française d'allergologie* reports the case of a woman treated for asthma who has a known allergy to dust mites, cats, and mugwort. After consuming cooked or raw ginger, her throat swelled and she had an asthma attack. Another woman, age fifty-nine, described trouble breathing or anaphylaxis on multiple occasions following the ingestion of medicinal plants containing ginger. The allergen responsible for these reactions is a cysteine protease known as GP-I. If you suspect you might have this kind of allergy, don't hesitate to consult an allergist who will be able to confirm this hypothesis with testing.

If you are considering using poppers—nitrite-based liquids that can be inhaled to "relax" before sex—you need to be aware that they have been known to cause tachycardia, migraines, nausea, and fainting, all of which are aggravated when taken alongside other medications. From an allergy standpoint, it is worth noting that cases of facial dermatitis linked to butyl nitrate have been reported over the years. Using these products to spice up your sex life can be dangerous, and everyone who uses them should be informed about the risks.

Moving on to something else, let's talk about **personal gel lubricants**. As their name implies, they're there to provide moisture, either during sex or in the battle against everyday vaginal dryness in menopausal women. Allergies to these products have been reported, so when you are choosing one make sure it does not contain any substances that you or your partner are allergic to: essential oils, fragrances, menthol, xanthan gum (E 415), phenoxyethanol, acrylates, etc. This will help you avoid any major surprises like eczema in the days following sex.

When we think of **piercings**, we usually picture a person's ears, tongue, eyebrow, nose, or navel. But some people take this idea even further and choose to affix these tiny adornments to their most private parts instead. In men, the most commonly pierced locations are the pubis, foreskin, the head of the penis, and the scrotum. Women tend to pierce the clitoris or vulva.

The problem with these piercings is that the jewelry may contain nickel, which is known to be highly allergenic. Be careful!

And while we're on the subject of accessories, remember that the primary ingredient in most **sex toys** is latex. The rubber accelerators in these pleasure objects can cause contact eczema, so if you're allergic to them, there will be swelling. And there will be itching. And if you're thinking of using a vegetable to be on the safe side, be warned that masturbating with a carrot has been reported to cause swelling of the vulva!

Kegel balls seem to have acquired a renewed following since the release of *Fifty Shades of Grey*. They have two very different functions. The first is pelvic floor rehabilitation to improve things like urinary incontinence, and the second is to tone vaginal muscles in order to achieve intense and unparalleled orgasms (the latter can be enhanced by the use of a remote control). Or at least that's what it says on the websites where they are sold. Centuries ago, these balls were made from precious and semi-precious stones, but silicon or metal make up the majority of what is available today. The exact composition is never really specified on the packaging or on the websites, so be mindful if you have a nickel or chromium allergy. Balls that feature bumps and ridges for extra pleasure may contain spandex and plastic. Depending on what you're allergic to, this could be important information. . . .

If you are more interested in **vibrators**, vibratory urticaria could pose a problem. This rare form of chronic hives (meaning symptoms last longer than six weeks) was first described in the

1970s. Just like other kinds of physical urticaria,* vibratory urticaria can be triggered by all kinds of different things, not just
sex! Any vibration, from a dildo to a bike ride, lawn mower, jack-
hammer, massage, sewing machine, or an electric razor could
trigger severe itching and red wheals that may be accompanied
by local swelling wherever the body was in contact with intense,
repeated vibrations. It may be a good idea to avoid this kind of
local stimulation!

At the end of our section on enhanced sexual sensation, it
is worth mentioning that male masturbation can cause hives of
its own known as "delayed pressure urticaria." Symptoms of this
condition include red spots on the penis and difficulty urinat-
ing for a few hours. This kind of physical urticaria following
prolonged pressure can also appear on the lips after a long and
passionate kiss!

Honeymoon rhinitis—*not* an allergy

Even though the clinical symptoms may look almost identical,
not all rhinitis is allergy-related. Let's take a closer look at this
somewhat odd condition.

In 2008, a physician published a fascinating case report.
His patient, a man, came to his first appointment with a rather
perplexing set of symptoms: whenever he had sexual thoughts,
he experienced violent fits of sneezing. The man had no known
ear-nose-throat or psychiatric pathology, and the doctor was not
sure what could be causing this until he found a similar problem

---

* Triggered by pressure or exposure to heat or cold.

mentioned in the 1870s. The possibility of a link between the nasal appendage and sexual arousal was evoked but without any explanation. In 1972, a man almost in his seventies was reported to experience rhinitis just after orgasm. Not many epidemiological studies have focused on this area, I must admit. Nevertheless, a few years later, a different group of doctors described roughly twenty patients with the same timeline of symptoms who complained of sneezing, runny nose, and congestion during the first five to fifteen minutes after sex.

The exact mechanism is not yet understood, but a pair of cranial nerves called the trigeminal nerves appear to play an essential role in triggering sneezes. Some scientists think these strange sex-related bouts of sneezing may be connected to "parasympathetic summation," which is when stimulation of one parasympathetic* nerve is accompanied by unexpected parasympathetic activity in other organs.

A few more recent articles have described this unique issue and sometimes refer to it as postcoital rhinitis or even postcoital asthma. In the 1990s, two researchers reported this problem in three men and one woman. In one of the patients, acute respiratory symptoms resulted in several trips to the emergency room followed by a hospitalization. The doctors ruled out exercise-induced asthma after a normal stress test including going up two

---

* The parasympathetic or vagal nervous system has a variety of functions such as lowering heart rate, aiding digestion, regulating our sphincters, contracting the pupil in response to light, and acting on the bronchial tree. It also plays a major role in sexual arousal.

flights of stairs.* They were left with the possibility that sexual arousal may have something to do with it. This kind of condition can often cause stress both for the person who experiences the symptoms and their partner, which can get in the way of a healthy sex life.

Keeping up appearances

When it comes to attracting a mate, human beings have a dizzying array of techniques at their disposal to help them look their best. But doing whatever it takes in the name of seduction doesn't always turn out the way we hoped, particularly when it comes to allergies.

Nail polish

Plenty of influencers on Instagram and TikTok inundate us with photographs of their incredibly long fake nails, but what they may not know is that those nails have the potential to send the person wearing them or applying them straight to the allergist's office.

Semipermanent polishes and artificial nails are primarily made from acrylates and methacrylates, so it shouldn't be much of a surprise that they are the cause of many cases of contact eczema in the nail area and on the face and eyelids where allergens present on the hands are most often deposited. The skin is very thin in these areas and therefore very sensitive.

---

* Equivalent to the effort of having sex.

Semipermanent polish is used in the form of a gel that hardens under ultraviolet light. The skin reactions mentioned above used to be limited to dental technicians who were in regular contact with acrylates and methacrylates because they are used in the construction of orthodontic appliances and some crowns. But now nail technicians are encountering similar problems including eczema on the hands and splitting fissures on the fingertips. Unfortunately, acrylates are very aggressive and can penetrate protective gloves.

Artificial nails contain the following resins that could cause allergies:

- Methyl methacrylate (MMA)
- 2-Hydroxyethyl methacrylate (2-HEMA)
- 2-hydroxypropyl methacrylate (2-HPMA)
- Ethylene glycol dimethacrylate (EGDMA)

Ethyl cyanoacrylate, which is used in nail and eyelash glue, is another irritant that should be added to the above list.

Waxing

Everyone has their preferred method for making hair in the pubic region disappear, and that's fine. If, however, a woman decides on a Brazilian bikini wax, certain things have to be kept in mind. This method is intended to remove most of a woman's pubic hair with the exception of a small "landing strip" or triangle above the vulva. A Hollywood wax, on the other hand, removes all hair in the intimate area. Regardless of whether or not you find this an attractive choice, anyone interested should know that it can cause irritation, inflammation, and that's not all. . . . Here are the ingredients in hot wax that people might be allergic to:

- Colophony (highly allergenic rosin)
- Lanolin (sheep's wool extract)
- Certain fragrances
- Beeswax

So, next time you're heading to get waxed, read up on the wax ingredients so you can make an informed decision before contact eczema turns your pubic region into something resembling a cauliflower.

If this intimate zone does happen to be hair-free, it may be tempting to try a vatoo, an airbrushed temporary tattoo, on the upper vaginal area. Again, as an allergist, I must warn you not to use these products. They are marketed as being henna-based but often contain PPD hair dye (also called p-diaminobenzene). The havoc wreaked by temporary tattoos with this product on other parts of the body should give you some idea about whether or not it's worth being careful. If you have had a problem with hair dye in the past, definitely avoid vatooing.

Eyebrow treatments

Until a certain female patient came to my office, I had never investigated this topic and I had certainly never heard of microblading. But since that was what had given her eczema on her forehead and eyebrows, I picked up my pilgrim's staff to go on a quest to find out more. Microblading is a semipermanent tattooing technique that gives the many women who have hopped on this bandwagon a more attractive eyebrow shape. Over the course of two appointments spaced one month apart, tiny needles are used to inject pigments (some of which contain PPD) beneath the skin. During this waiting period is often when disaster strikes for allergy sufferers. Within days, this procedure can trigger a severe case of contact eczema in the injected area and, worst of all, these pigments cannot be removed! As early as twenty-four to forty-eight hours after a microblading session, people may experience itching and redness followed by a cascade of less than glamorous symptoms including papules, vesicles, oozing blisters, and local swelling. If the area becomes infected—which can happen—then it's time for treatment with corticosteroids and antibiotics. Allergy patch testing can be performed a few weeks or months after the acute reaction.

Some women prefer tinting the hair on their eyebrows instead of microblading, but even this can cause such severe swelling of the eyelids that a few days later they can barely open their eyes.

We know that PPD may be an ingredient in hair dyes and temporary tattoos that purport to be henna-based, but if you are allergic to PPD you may also react to substances like azo dyes that are present in other coloring products. Here are a few azo dyes that are known to cause allergic reactions:

- Toluene-2,5-diamine
- P-aminophenol
- 2-nitro-PPD
- Disperse orange dyes

Fragrances

The intoxicating scent of a perfume or cologne does seem to work a sort of come-hither magic in the dance of sexual attraction, and a beautifully scented room certainly helps everyone get in the mood, but these products also contain a multitude of allergens that can trigger severe contact eczema flare-ups. Room sprays, in fact, have even been known to provoke asthma attacks.

25 Fragrance Allergens Subject to Individual Labeling in the European Union*

Alpha-Isomethyl ionone	Synthetic
Amyl cinnamal	Synthetic
Amyl cinnamyl alcohol	Synthetic
Anise alcohol	Synthetic or natural: essential oils of anise, Tahiti vanilla
Benzyl alcohol	Synthetic or natural: Peru balsam, Tolu balsam, jasmine essential oil
Benzyl benzoate	Synthetic or natural: Peru balsam, Tolu balsam, essential oils of jasmine or ylang-ylang
Benzyl cinnamate	Synthetic or natural: Peru balsam, Copahu, Tolu balsam
Benzyl salicylate	Synthetic or natural: propolis
Butylphenyl methylpropional	Synthetic
Cinnamal	Synthetic or natural: essential oils of cinnamon, hyacinth, patchouli

(Continued on next page)

Cinnamyl alcohol	Synthetic or natural: hyacinth
Citral	Synthetic or natural: essential oils of lemon, orange peel, mandarin orange, or eucalyptus
Citronellol	Synthetic or natural: Ceylon citronella essential oil
Coumarin	Synthetic or natural: woodruff, sweet vernal grass, sweet clover, angelica, giant hogweed
Eugenol	Synthetic or natural: essential oils of clove, allspice, bay, avens, Ceylon cinnamon, laurel, cistus, basil, sassafras, Java basil, cassie, sweet flag, carnation, boldo, cascarilla, galangal, bay leaves, nutmeg, pale rose, ylang-ylang, marjoram, camphor, lemongrass, patchouli
Farnesol	Synthetic or natural: essential oils of rose, neroli, ylang-ylang, lime tree, Tolu balsam
Geraniol	Synthetic or natural: essential oils of rose, orange, palmarosa, thyme, verbena, neroli, lemongrass, geranium, hyssop, laurel, lavender, mandarin orange, melissa, nutmeg, myrtle
Hexyl cinnamal	Synthetic
Hydroxycitronnellal	Synthetic
Isoeugenol	Synthetic or natural: essential oils of lemongrass, Ceylon, ylang-ylang
Limonene	Synthetic or natural: essential oils of lemon, dill, common juniper, orange, verbena, neroli, niaouli, melaleuca, melissa, peppermint, nutmeg, myrrh, angelica, lavender aspic, star anise, bergamot, mandarin, bitter orange, caraway, celery, lavender, lime
Linalool	Synthetic or natural: essential oils of thyme, lavender, pine, laurel, bitter orange, marjoram, peppermint, lemon, orange, ylang-ylang, verbena, myrtle, neroli, coriander, geranium, lime, melissa, nutmeg, lemongrass, basil, bergamot, rosewood
Methyl 2-octynoate	Synthetic
Evernia prunastri (Oak moss)	Natural: oak moss extract
Evernia furfuracea (Tree moss)	Natural: tree moss extract

The FDA uses the European Union's list as a reference.

Fillers

Staying young is, naturally, the unspoken wish of a great many people. Fillers can help, but are they free of allergy risks?

Hyaluronic acid fillers treat signs of aging while other kinds like cross-linked hyaluronic acid, calcium hydroxylapatite, and poly-L-lactic acid are used to "sculpt" the skin of the face.

These products are classified as medical devices in the United States, but this is not a guarantee against harmful side effects. Injections should only be given by a medical professional who has been trained to administer these products and should always be preceded by a medical exam and interview to eliminate any of the following risk factors: autoimmune disease, interferon treatment, omalizumab treatment, chronic herpes, and the use of other medications such as anticoagulants.

Hyaluronic acid breaks down in the body within six to twelve months, whereas the effects of poly-L-lactic acid and calcium hydroxylapatite last for around two years.

Beware of fillers containing non-biodegradables like acrylates or alkylamides. Because of their sometimes severe and delayed side effects (ten to twenty years later in some cases), fillers containing silicone are illegal in some countries.

Allergic reactions to fillers are rare and their mechanism can be immediate or delayed. Symptoms may include the appearance of granulomas or local inflammation. Hyaluronic acid is usually well-tolerated, but all precautionary measures should be respected.

Society today revolves around social success, the illusion or reality of a flourishing sex life, and boundless youth, which sometimes leaves little room for people to talk about what they're really going through, especially when it comes to the bedroom. Allergies that affect intimacy deserve to be taken into consideration more often so that everyone has the chance to thrive and enjoy sex.

PART TWO

ALLERGY RIDDLES
AND CURIOSITIES

A Note from Alex Dessinateur

As cartoonists, we're used to getting all kinds of requests—sometimes they're work-related (for press or media relations) and other times people ask for something more personal. Those are usually the funnier ones, actually. So I can't say that I was surprised to get an email from Catherine. I already knew she was a fan of my cartoons in the *Courrier Picard*. What I was not expecting was the surprising proposition that her email contained!

Catherine said she was in the process of writing a book about allergies (nothing abnormal about that—she's an allergist, after all), and even though we had never met, she informed me that she wanted me to write the introduction. . . .

For a few seconds I thought she must have sent the email to the wrong person by mistake. But then I noticed her references to my illustrations. But why would a scientist want a few lines penned by her professional opposite, someone with no expertise whatsoever in the field of allergy medicine? I love a good mismatch, and I'd certainly been given one! And, if I'm honest, it did feel somewhat relevant to my own life because I was allergic to cats as a child. As soon as I went near a feline, my face would immediately look like a myxomatosis-riddled version of the worst caricatures to ever appear out of my pen. This allergy disappeared thirty years later when I adopted an adorable little kitten who showed up at my house without any invitation. I have to confess that my children didn't leave me much of a choice. Had psychology somehow come into play here? Was I now immune to contact with my epidermal enemy? Meeting Catherine confirmed for me that humor and medicine are not necessarily antonyms. I found myself in the presence of someone who is passionate about what she does and fascinating to listen to. I also learned all about the allergy/immunology specialty, one that has only recently been made trendy by hipster gluten exterminators who would wipe their enemy off the face of the earth if they could! My apologies—that was clearly a caricature. A cartoonist's occupational hazard, I suppose. . . .

What I discovered in this book completely stupefied, captivated, and amazed me. These scientific discoveries, which one could easily dismiss as highly embellished hearsay, will literally transport you to a world that is so unknown it deserves a Hollywood movie—and I say this knowing that most of the characters would be busy itching and sniffling through most of their lines!

I found myself utterly immersed in Catherine Quéquet's medical detective work, and I can guarantee, reader, that you have no idea what surprises are in store for you in these pages. Every story she tells is like a cartoon slowly taking shape on a blank page: the first lines intrigue you, and then you have no idea how it's all going to end until the last drop of ink has found its place. Are you allergic to science and humor? No? Wonderful, because both are good for your health!

CHAPTER 6

Who's the Culprit?

We've seen how important it is to examine the timeline leading up to an allergic reaction and to firmly ground any diagnosis in the results of allergy testing—now let's play a little game. It's time for you to be the detective and unmask what's causing the allergy! I think you're going to see why every piece of information in a story absolutely *must* be taken into account.

Riddles

The lovely Élise

Élise is in her thirties, very active, and a real fashionista. Every day she posts stories about fashion on her Instagram, and her followers love her outfits and beauty suggestions. Her goal? To become a famous influencer.

I have to hand it to her—she does know what she's talking about when it comes to hair and makeup. As a teenager, Élise dreamed of only one thing: owning her own hair salon. She started a vocational training course but left without finishing the program. During her internship at a salon, she noticed small bumps gradually appearing all over her palms. After a few days, the itching became unbearable and her fingers were covered in blisters. It was truly hell. The local treatments her doctor prescribed didn't help, and she had to stop working for several weeks. At an emergency consultation with an allergist, the doctor mentioned the possibility of a work-related allergy. Tests performed at the allergist's office confirmed this hypothesis. The verdict was in: Élise would never be able to become a hairdresser. The guilty party is that darn PPD used in dark hair dyes. Crushed, the young girl changed directions and decided to try a career in selling ready-to-wear clothing.

One thing led to another, and thanks to social media, Élise started forming connections with other people on the platform. This is when she started thinking about becoming an influencer. This is also how she met and fell for David, a young man with everything she usually looks for: he plays four sports and has a beard, and he's also tall, brown-haired, and a little bit of a hipster. They lived around sixty miles apart, but that didn't discourage them, and they met up as soon as they could.

Ever since she started seeing David a few weeks ago, Élise has been having skin problems on her face and abdomen. The dry red patches on her cheeks and chin flare up now and then and itch day and night. This is not a very easy time for her, and posting on Instagram with red spots all over her face is, of course, completely out of the question. She goes back to her allergist. The doctor asks her what cosmetic products she uses and about her daily habits. Has she had any additional exposure to PPD since her adolescence? The young woman admits that she did bend the rules once two or three years ago when she couldn't resist getting a temporary tattoo on vacation. The appearance of eczema at the site two days later made her bitterly regret her choice—the tattoo she received must have been a mixture of natural henna and PPD. Apart from that incident she has strictly respected her doctor's orders.

The allergist tests all of her cosmetics as well as other products in the European standard allergen battery. Apart from PPD, which is still positive, no other allergens cause a reaction. So where are these patches coming from? Who's the culprit?

See solution on page 161

The two brothers

Thomas and Mathieu are brothers born a few years apart. One has allergies, the other does not. Thomas has a peanut allergy that requires management on a daily basis. For almost thirteen years he has reacted to even the slightest trace of this legume in his food. The slightest contact could be fatal. Everyone at school is aware of the danger and a special protocol has been in place for years. Luckily, the boy is also very sensible. Friends and family all know—not one peanut or peanut-flavored cookie or cracker can cross the threshold of the house. His older brother, Mathieu, has always lived with his brother's allergy in the back of his mind. Sometimes, though, he wishes he didn't have to.

The last time Thomas had accidental contact with peanuts, the reaction was extremely severe. His face quickly started swelling and he had trouble breathing. He even vomited. Fortunately, the onset of anaphylaxis was cut short by a rapid injection of epinephrine in his thigh. He was monitored for several hours in a hospital and everything turned out just fine.

The family used to live in an apartment where the two boys had bunk beds in the same room. Now they live in a larger house and each brother has his own bedroom. Two bedrooms, two very different ambiances. Thomas, the younger brother, is more of a geek. He's usually playing video games or using the new laptop computer his grandparents recently bought for him. Mathieu is a handsome and athletic seventeen-year-old who is already successful with the ladies. He has a computer in his room, too, but sometimes he borrows his brother's. Mathieu's bedroom is not a model of organization. His mother is always scolding him about it but there's not much she can do. And when his friends come over to spend the afternoon in what they call his "cave," it doesn't exactly help matters.

Just about every Saturday, Pierre, Manu, Louis, Amandine, and Sarah come to the house and hunker down in Mathieu's room. Thomas has complained two or three times about them borrowing his laptop. And then there was that terrible Sunday. Thomas had gone to take his computer back once again from his brother's room. He started typing on the keyboard and his voice instantly changed and became hoarse. He felt nauseated, his eyelids became swollen, and his face and hands were suddenly covered in hives. But he hadn't eaten anything for several hours and hadn't seen a peanut in years! He didn't understand, and neither did his parents. They rushed into his room when they heard his frightened screams, and his mother injected him with epinephrine while his father called an ambulance. Thomas spent the next few hours being monitored at the hospital. So, what happened to cause Thomas to have an allergic reaction?

See solution on page 162

You don't have to be the Hulk

Nicolas is twenty years old and thinks he's a little too skinny. He has always been bothered by his slender frame. At school people called him "the beanpole." Now he's decided to take matters into his own hands. His first investment in this process involves the purchase of some nifty workout clothes. The unspoken reason for this transformation is clearly the sweet and beautiful Lucie, a petite blonde with green eyes who Nicolas really likes. Once he's signed up at a gym, he starts his training program. He sweats, suffering in silence, going from one machine to another. The motivation is there, but so are the muscle cramps. His friends encourage him to keep going, and his body starts to build muscle. Nicolas feels much better about himself. His body is doing more than usual and sometimes he feels a little tired, but he won't give up. As the weeks go by, he becomes friends with other gym members. Sweating together two or three times a week does bring people closer. Everyone encourages one another. Marco, a longtime bodybuilder, always has advice to give. One day, he tells Nicolas that spirulina supplements could help him build muscle mass and increase his endurance. Ever the good student, Nicolas obeys and buys a container of this supposedly miraculous product. Everything might have worked out wonderfully had it not been for that dark Thursday . . .

Just like every day, the young man has breakfast at 7:30. He quickly gobbles down an apple, cereal, a coffee, and a slice of buttered bread, accompanied by four spirulina tablets. But today, Nicolas won't make it to the gym. Five hours later, his body is covered in hives. His eyelids swell and he has pain when he swallows. He feels like something is really wrong, and his reflex to call emergency medical services is what saves his life. His symptoms were actually the beginnings of an anaphylactic reaction. Nicolas is told not to consume any of the things he ingested the day of the episode. He has no known food allergies, and this is confirmed by a specialized round of testing a few months later. So what happened?

See solution on page 165

One baby, two pistols?

Inès is an adorable five-month-old baby girl. This little blondie with azure eyes and long eyelashes is the joy of her whole family. Her father, Bertrand, is a big guy but melts for his little princess, and Lisa, her mother, is a pretty woman in her thirties who devotes most of her time to taking care of the girl. Soon, though, she'll have to go back to work. Mrs. X, the nanny, will step in. In this fantasy, the baby's grandparents are always around, and happily so. For the moment, the baby has no allergies. Grandma Malou had been a little worried because her daughter Lisa had been allergic to cow's milk proteins as a baby before growing out of the allergy at the age of four. She was afraid the same thing would happen to her granddaughter.

The little girl is in perfect health until the day the nanny starts seeing small red spots and very dry skin in the diaper area. Nothing alarming, but she still decides to tell the parents. "It's strange," she says, "the spots are only on the sides. Diaper rash is usually on the baby's bottom." Days pass and the skin problems get worse. Blisters appear. No cream can calm the baby's symptoms, and even the doctor is at a loss. Corticosteroids in small quantities help a little, but the problem always comes back. The baby starts getting fussy. She scratches herself with her chubby little fingers. The irritation is still in the same place—on both hips and outer thighs, with nothing on her abdomen or her bottom. What in the world is going on?

See solution on page 166

Solutions
The lovely Élise

David takes care of himself. His beard is actually a little gray, but Élise doesn't know that. He is too embarrassed to admit to her that he dyes it with a product containing PPD. Like other cases we've seen, this is an example of a consort allergy or contact allergy by proxy.

PPD is found in temporary tattoos—I'll say it again, these are not worth the blisters, pustules, and lesions that could ruin your life within forty-eight hours and last several weeks if you don't get them treated—as well as hair dyes and dyes for beards and eyebrows. A contact allergy by proxy did not appear to be the obvious culprit at first, but thanks to a meticulous investigation the allergen was tracked down and eventually identified, on the partner in this case.

The two brothers

When the older brother had friends over on Saturday, at around 6:00 p.m. they made themselves a little something to eat. The boys had brought beer. Sarah and Amandine had packed salted peanuts and other snacks. They had totally forgotten about his little brother's allergy. For once, Mathieu doesn't see a problem because they're in his bedroom. His little brother isn't there. As usual, his sidekicks eventually go and get the laptop from Thomas's bedroom. The peanut allergens on their sticky fingers are deposited on the keyboard. This is why when Thomas is playing on his laptop the next day, the peanut allergens trigger a severe reaction via skin contact.

This story is based on the following case, which was described in 2006 in the *Revue française d'allergologie*. A nine-year-old boy was taken to see an allergist after something rather unusual happened. At a family dinner, the child had had an allergic reaction to peanuts despite the fact that he hadn't eaten any. He had been quietly playing video games. After a thorough investigation, it turns out that his uncle, a gamer, had used the boy's PlayStation after eating peanut-flavored corn puffs and other snacks. Without realizing it, the adult had deposited peanut allergens on the game controls, which triggered hives and facial swelling when his nephew came into contact with them. Luckily, everything returned to normal after the boy was treated with prednisolone and cetirizine.

I found this kind of reaction caused by accidental exposure in another article, too. This time the victim was a thirty-two-year-old man with a peanut allergy. During a card game with three other people, he started having difficulty breathing and his lips and tongue began to swell. The other players had been careful to eat their peanuts in another room, but when they came back to finish the game they didn't wash their hands and the peanut proteins on their fingers were deposited onto the cards. Before dealing, our "victim" licked his thumb to help separate the cards, thereby making contact with the allergen, which rapidly set off his symptoms.

For anyone with a food allergy, knowing how to avoid "cross-contact" with an allergen is extremely important. Cross-contact simply means that an allergen is present on a surface where it shouldn't be. This can be in the home, as we just saw, but it can also occur during manufacturing when a small amount of an allergenic food accidentally comes into contact with another food product and "contaminates" it.

People with food allergies should also avoid getting their fresh bread sliced at the bakery. The bread that was in the slicer before your loaf may have contained nuts, and those allergens will likely have been deposited onto the slicer's blades. The same goes for sliced meats purchased from a butcher or deli—if the butcher just sliced up some mortadella with pistachios, how can you be certain no allergens were left behind?

A recent study on the persistence of peanut allergen on table surfaces concluded that the allergen Ara h 1 can remain on an uncleaned table surface for 110 days. When dealing with such a "robust" allergen, which cleaning products are best? According to this same study:

- Dish soap: potential persistence of allergen residue—NO.
- Alcohol-based hand sanitizer also left allergens behind on the scrubbed surface—NO.
- YES for liquid soaps and bar soaps with water (soapy water).
- Hand wipes can also help eradicate food allergens from flat surfaces, but you still have to deal with the risk of a contact allergy.
- The sponge used to clean a surface may have allergens on it—be careful.

If you're concerned about cross-contact during food manufacturing—and rightly so!—you should know that Hazard Analysis Critical Control Point (HACCP) is available to help prevent that. Food manufacturers can use this approach to make sure their products will not harm consumers.

To ensure safety, HACCP follows seven key principles:

1. Analysis of potential allergy risk due to accidental cross-contact (hazard analysis).
2. Identification of critical control points (the presence of an allergen not in the initial recipe and therefore not indicated on the packaging).
3. Establish critical limits (what is the maximum amount of allergen that can safely be present?).
4. Establish monitoring procedures.
5. Establish corrective actions (when the critical limit is too high, for example, unsafe food may have to be removed from the market).
6. Establish verification procedures to make sure the HACCP method is effective.
7. Establish record-keeping and documentation procedures.

You don't have to be the Hulk

Spirulina was the culprit.

The first case of this allergy was reported in 2010. A thirteen-year-old boy broke out in hives and developed swollen upper eyelids six hours after ingesting five spirulina tablets. After a short hospitalization and the appropriate treatment, he was fine. A few weeks later, allergy testing confirmed that spirulina had caused his reaction. In 2014, the French Agency for Food,

Environmental and Occupational Health & Safety (ANSES) published a warning regarding an identical case in 2011. A thirty-five-year-old man had started taking two spoonsful of spirulina a day to help boost his energy levels. After three days, he experienced rhinitis symptoms with difficulty breathing, hives, and swollen eyelids. He was treated for the reaction and allergy testing confirmed a spirulina allergy—the allergen to blame was phycocyanin.

There are several kinds of blue-green microalgae on the market, but the one most often used as a food supplement is *Arthrospira platensis*, which comes in powder, gel, or tablet form. Most people take it as a treatment for muscle cramps and to reduce fatigue. Spirulina is also rich in protein (60 percent) and vitamin B12 and often appears in vegetarian meals.

One baby, two pistols?

Little Inès is experiencing what experts refer to as "Lucky Luke" dermatitis.

This form of contact eczema is a fairly unusual skin problem observed in infants. The skin reaction is localized to the outer buttocks and hips, exactly where a cowboy's holsters would sit, hence the name.

First described in 1998, Lucky Luke dermatitis develops after sensitization to rubber components in disposable diapers like mercaptobenzothiazole and cyclohexylthiophthalimide. P-tert-butylphenol formaldehyde resin used in the diaper's adhesive can cause the same problem. If allergy tests for these chemicals are negative, some researchers believe this reaction should be considered a symptom of atopic eczema if the infant has a family history of allergies.

This should under no circumstances be confused with the typical diaper rash the nanny in the story described. The latter causes painful skin lesions on the baby's buttocks and genitals, lower abdomen, and upper thighs without involvement of skin folds.

CHAPTER 7

The Question-and-Answer Game

For years now, I've been writing quizzes on social media. I think learning something new in a fun way and online is as good a way as any to commit that information to memory. Here are a few quiz questions for you. Take a stab at them and see what you learn!

Questions

Something smells fishy

If a person is allergic to fish, are they taking a risk walking around a fish market even if they don't touch or eat anything?

1. Yes.
2. Oh no, not at all.
3. I don't know.

Hive mentality

It's winter and lots of people are tempted to reinforce their immune systems by eating honey or royal jelly (even though this has no proven immune benefits). There's no harm in it, so why not? On the other hand, you need to be especially careful if you're allergic to:

1. Mold.
2. Pollen.
3. Bee stings (wasp, bumblebee, hornet).

Strange worms

A young man has small cracks on the thumb and index finger of both hands as well as his right middle finger. This is not work-related and the fissures only appear when he is on vacation. The skin around his nails is severely inflamed. He enjoys running races, but his favorite leisure activity is fishing. What is the cause of his skin issues? Contact with:

1. The fishing pole.
2. Fish.
3. Maggots.

Like the Amish

In which community are people more likely to have asthma, the Indiana Amish or the South Dakota Hutterites?

1. The Amish, because of their horse-drawn buggies and traditional way of life.

2. The Hutterites, who use more modern and mechanized farming techniques.

Pain in my pumps

Mrs. X has a big problem—the soles of her feet are covered in blisters and dry patches. Everywhere except her arches. She rides horses and wears sneakers or leather shoes most of the time. What is causing her reaction?

1. Chrome-tanned leather.
2. Mercaptobenzothiazole, a rubber accelerator.

Chicken and aquatic animals

If someone is allergic to chicken, he or she may also react to:

1. Fish.
2. Amphibians.
3. Crocodile meat.

Answers

Something smells fishy

The correct answer is 1.

Walking around stalls of seafood in open or covered markets is not the best idea if you have a fish allergy. According to medical literature on this topic, the very smell of fish can trigger a reaction. For people predisposed to allergies, the allergenic particles of raw fish floating in the air can also pose a hazard and provoke symptoms like eczema flare-ups, asthma attacks, or even anaphylaxis. A medical journal article published in 2017 describes the case of a young boy whose face broke out in hives when he and his mother arrived at the fishmonger. He started sneezing and developed a runny nose, his eyes reddened, and he had difficulty breathing.

Fish allergies affect 0.1–3 percent of the general population, with a more marked frequency in Scandinavian countries, Japan, and Spain, all of which are large fish consumers. According to the FDA, in the United States fish is third on the list of major food allergens, and according to FoodAllergy.org, 40 percent of people with fish allergies don't experience their first reactions until adulthood. The least allergenic fish is tuna and mackerel.

Fish allergens belong to the parvalbumin family and are typically concentrated in the fish's head and white muscle meat. These proteins are thermoresistant and therefore not destroyed by cooking. They can also be inhaled in cooking vapors.

For professionals like fishmongers and wholesalers, inhaling fish allergens can result in sensitization. In 2000, a team of physicians in Madrid collected air samples from fish markets over a period of forty-one days. Other samples were taken from outdoor residential areas. The results were startling: allergenic proteins were present in high levels at the fish markets but were completely absent from the residential areas.

What is true of these seafood products is true of other foods. Food allergen exposure (causing an allergic reaction or a potential sensitization) can happen:

- If an odor or cooking vapor is inhaled.
- If an allergenic food is touched with the hands.
- While fruits and vegetables are being peeled.

Take, for instance, the case of a twenty-five-year-old nurse with a milk allergy who had trouble breathing and an asthma attack at a dairy farm. Dr. Paul Molkhou reported this case in a journal article and provided the additional example of a shepherd allergic to cow's milk who had an asthma attack while milking his sheep.

Hive mentality
The right answer is 2.
People with pollen allergies are advised not to eat beehive products or dietary supplements containing pollen they are allergic to. In France, for example, the surge in severe allergic reactions observed after ingesting products like royal jelly and propolis prompted the French Agency for Food, Environmental and Occupational Health & Safety (ANSES) to publish recommendations on their website in July 2018.

Honey flavor varies depending on what plant the bees have been foraging in. In the United States, there are more than three hundred unique types of honey available. Bees (*Apis mellifera*) make honey from flower nectar or from honeydew excreted by plant suckers like aphids after they have digested plant sap. The composition of a particular honey varies by season and the geographic location of the beehives.

Since ancient times, honey has had a variety of uses, most notably in the domains of medicine and cosmetics.

The first observation of a honey allergy was recorded in 1984. A forty-two-year-old beekeeper with a known allergy to mugwort, chamomile, and dandelion pollen had an allergic reaction after eating honey containing this kind of pollen. She had previously eaten honey she produced herself without any problems because it did not contain pollen from these plants. A few publications since then have reported similar findings.

A medical team from Marseille described a similar case in France in 1989. A fifty-year-old beekeeper was treated with epinephrine and corticosteroids for anaphylaxis a few minutes after consuming sunflower honey. He had known for several years that he was allergic to celery. A microscopic analysis of the honey he consumed revealed the following composition: 12 percent sunflower pollen, 83 percent chestnut pollen, 4 percent Rosaceae pollen, and 1 percent composites. Skin tests were positive for ragweed, mugwort, sunflower, daisy, and dandelion. Remember that an allergy to mugwort pollen can cause cross-reactivity with celery.

Since then, more than a few cases have been reported of anaphylaxis after ingestion of honey containing several kinds of pollen. Each time the victim had a history of pollen allergy. The clinical symptoms are identical to symptoms of an IgE-mediated food allergy reaction: hives, swelling, digestive trouble with abdominal pain and diarrhea, and asthma attacks.

Note

Honey is a fascinating blend of nectar, propolis, pollen allergens, and proteins secreted by specialized glands in the bee's body. Interestingly, it is possible to be allergic to honey without also having pollen allergies. This allergy, in fact, is the cause of symptoms in 17percent of people who experience digestive issues. In 2017, the *Revue française d'allergologie* reported the case of a man who had been experiencing chronic diarrhea for several years. He ate honey with his breakfast every day. On occasion he also consumed royal jelly, which would usually lead to angioedema thirty minutes later. As soon as he stopped eating these products, the diarrhea totally disappeared. Since he was not allergic to pollen, this proves that the allergy was in fact to the honey itself. The allergens responsible for these kinds of honey allergies are called major royal jelly proteins.

Honey and traces of it may be ingredients in manufactured food products like frozen french fries, chips, vinegar, nougat, gingerbread, etc.

Royal jelly is secreted by worker bees between their fifth and fourteenth day of life to nourish the larvae and the queen bee. We humans consume it in the form of capsules, ampoules, or liquid for its supposed immune system benefits. Allergic reactions to royal jelly are usually severe immediately and include acute asthma attacks, significant swelling, or anaphylaxis, particularly if the victim has an atopic family history or known bee sting allergies.

Bee pollen granules are said to have stimulating and reparative effects on the body, but they can also trigger food allergies if someone is allergic to pollen.

Bees collect the raw ingredients to make **propolis** from the buds of certain trees and then mix it into wax to seal any holes in the hive. It contains (in decreasing order of concentration): resin, wax, aromatic oils, pollen, and other substances like vanillin or cinnamic aldehyde. This substance is known to cause contact eczema, the first case of which was recorded in the 1930s. In the world of cosmetics, propolis is used to make toothpaste, shampoo, lipstick, soap, and sunscreen, among other things.

Allergies to beehive products do not discriminate, and certain food industry workers are particularly susceptible (honey-based cereal manufacturers, honey extraction plant employees). These patients typically present with a respiratory allergy by inhalation that is categorized as occupational asthma.

"Melliferous plants are plants that produce the nectar that bees in a colony then transform into honey, but in a broader sense this name could apply to any plant that produces a substance that is useful to bees: an abundance of pollen, honeydew left on softwoods in the feces of aphids and ladybugs, and propolis."
—Dominique Gaudefroy, botanist

The CDC, as well as the French Agency for Food, Environmental and Occupational Health & Safety (ANSES), advises against the consumption of honey for children under the age of one. Since 2004, there has been a surge in infant botulism, which can lead to respiratory distress and hospitalization. How could this be connected to honey consumption? Bees may be carrying fragments of *Clostridium botulinum* that are then incorporated into the honey and, unfortunately, the immune system before age one is not yet mature enough to defend itself against this bacteria.

The ingestion of *Clostridium botulinum* spores contained in honey triggers the production of botulism toxin in the infant's digestive tract. Fairly quickly this leads to constipation, paralysis of the eye muscles, and loss of muscle tone that can make the child resemble a rag doll. In the event of respiratory distress, intubation and ventilation may be necessary. Infant botulism is a notifiable disease. The first case observed was in the United States in 1976. *Clostridium botulinum* spores resist heat and are not destroyed by boiling.

Many countries warn families about this problem and in some places it is even mentioned on the honey label.

Strange worms

Answer 3 is exactly right.

This is actually a case of contact eczema caused by proteins in the worms the man touches while fishing.* He always uses the first three fingers of his right hand to hold the worm and place it on the fish hook in his left hand and has noticed that whenever he comes home from fishing, his fingers are always swollen. Then, later, the skin on his fingertips starts cracking. Skin tests looking for the usual contact eczema suspects are all negative. Prick tests for red and white maggots, however, are positive.

---

* Published in the *Revue française d'allergologie*.

The name given to this skin condition is "protein contact dermatitis." It is often underdiagnosed and tends to affect food handlers (restaurant, bakery, and catering employees) and in particular individuals who work with animal meat (butchers, cooks, sausage makers, abattoir staff). The appearance of this condition is strongly linked to contact with proteins in fruits, legumes, spices, wood, plants, animals, seeds, and enzymes. Instead of hives, however, this dermatitis manifests in the form of chronic eczema. The acute flare-ups follow the pattern of contact with the allergen on the hands (fingers), wrists, and forearms, or—when the offending protein is floating through the air, like flour in a bakery, for example—on the face and neck.

As shown in an article from 2013, even professionals like hairdressers can be impacted by this allergy. A young woman, age seventeen, was training to be a hairdresser while completing other studies on the side. Her time was split between classes and internships in various salons. During these internships she was in daily contact with a range of products including shampoo, hair dye, and scalp masks. She had been noticing eczema on her hands for several months.

Usually, allergies in this professional setting are linked to PPD, persulfates in bleaching products, shampoo fragrance, or nickel in scissors.

For this young lady, though, all of the tests for these potential allergens were negative. The medical team decided to go a step further and began looking for an allergen that may have slipped into a product like a hair mask. They performed additional tests with four of these masks. Three of them were positive within twenty minutes. The cause of the intern's protein contact dermatitis was hydrolyzed keratin. Similar hair repair products may also contain wheat or oat proteins.

> **Classic contact eczema:** eczema appears after several days (delayed allergy). Allergens identified via patch tests.
> **Protein contact dermatitis:** eczema appears within twenty minutes (immediate allergy). Allergens identified via prick tests.

Like the Amish
The correct answer is the Hutterites.

The Hutterite religious community has seen the frequency of asthma in their school-age children quadruple. They also have a higher rate of infant asthma than the Amish (21.3 percent versus 5 percent) even though the way of life in the two communities is just about identical. The Hutterites, however, use more modern agricultural techniques, including farm machinery. Their environment is also more sanitized than that of the Indiana Amish, which can facilitate the development of this disease. The Amish are still anchored in more ancestral farming methods and use horses both for daily errands and in the fields. In 2017, a group of researchers studied asthma rates in the two populations and found that the difference could be explained by the contents of the dust in their respective living spaces. The dust in Amish country is rich in microbes. The authors of the study specify, of course, that the homes were well-maintained and clean and that this is not an indication that Amish homes are dirty!

In 2015, Belgian scientists observed that repeatedly exposing mice to bacterial endotoxins and low doses of viruses—or exposing them to farm dust every day—prevented them from developing asthma and allergies. The bronchial mucus membrane became less reactive to allergens like dust mites thanks to an A20 protein (a powerful anti-inflammatory discovered in mice) that the body produced when in contact with the farm dust.

These findings reinforce the theory that overcleaning favors the appearance of allergies and suggest that children who grow up in a microbe-rich agricultural environment surrounded by animals are less likely to have allergies and develop asthma.

As the granddaughter of a farmer, I can confirm that being close to nature has many benefits. Children find such joy in feeding rabbits, running after chickens, or walking around the stables. The same cannot be said for the cemented and soulless farms where the animals never see the light of day. But I digress.

Another team of researchers has offered an additional explanation for the lower allergy rates in children living in rural areas. Unlike other mammals, humans do not possess the enzyme CMP-Neu5Ac hydroxylase (CMAH). We are, as a result, incapable of producing Neu5Gc (N-glycolylneuraminic acid). When we are exposed to Neu5Gc, our immune system defends itself by producing anti-Neu5Gc antibodies. A European study called PARSIFAL took this information and decided to examine what causes infant asthma and allergies in farming families across five countries: Austria, the Netherlands, Germany, Sweden, and

Switzerland. The data they collected show that environmental exposure to Neu5Gc through contact with animals is associated with a lower frequency of asthma, though the exact mechanism is not yet understood. Once again, the microbial diversity in a child's environment appears to be the key protective factor in the development of an immune system that is not prone to allergies.

Pain in my pumps

The correct answer is mercaptobenzothiazole, a rubber accelerator.

This woman's shoes have a foam rubber insole, and the problem is localized to the soles of her feet. These lesions are most likely caused by a combination of heavy sweating and rubbing of her skin against the insole. Chrome-tanned leather is not the culprit because she does not have any problems on her heels or the sides of her feet.

Shoe contact eczema is responsible for 3–11 percent of skin allergy consultations. Symptoms are often bilateral and mirror the shape of the shoe on the skin. These range from dry skin to weeping sores, bumps, blisters, redness, and ulceration . . . not to mention furious itching, pain, and burning that sometimes makes it difficult to walk. Flare-ups may be acute or chronic, and this can determine how the contact eczema evolves over time.

The materials responsible for this reaction are many and varied:

- Leather, if it is tanned using trivalent chromium salts.
- Certain dyes.

- Adhesives like p-tert-butylphenol formaldehyde resin, colophony (also contained in shoe polish).
- Biocides like isothiazolinone and formaldehyde.

One particularly infamous anti-fungal called dimethyl fumarate caused quite a stir between 2006 and 2008. Do you remember the deep burns inflicted by shoes and sofas that had been manufactured in China and treated with this chemical? It was outlawed in Europe in 2009, but be on the lookout! It surreptitiously reappeared in northern France in July 2017, and the customer involved quickly regretted her purchase. Within a few hours of wearing her new shoes, she saw blisters and ulcerations appear on the soles of her feet.

If someone reacts to shoes made from natural rubber, additives like thiurams (a rubber vulcanization accelerator) are probably the cause.

Shoes made with plastic-based materials or synthetic rubber are manufactured using polyurethane or neoprene. Recently, a new compound called DMTBS (dimethylthiocarbamylbenzothiazole sulfide) has also appeared. Yes, that's the name, and saying it is enough to make you sneeze! DMTBS, often used in boat shoes, forms during the rubber manufacturing process. Cross-reactivity with thiurams is possible. I should also mention that neoprene is often incriminated in skin reactions to water shoes used for kayaking, diving, and sailing.

Next up on the list of potential troublemakers is (hold on to your hats!) 2-(thiocyanomethylthio) benzothiazole, an antifungal used in leather and faux leather shoes.

I'll end this section with a little nod to those of you who love flip-flops. If you suddenly see large blisters or bubbles on your feet, the evil villain is acetophenone azine, which is found in shin guards and in the ethylene-vinyl acetate foam used to make your much-loved sandals.

Chicken and aquatic animals

In fact, all three answers are correct.

The reason for this is simple: a common protein called parvalbumin. As we saw in a previous case, fish allergies are caused by proteins in the parvalbumin family. This protein is also found:

- In amphibians, which explains why there is a risk of allergic reaction when eating frogs.
- In gallinaceous birds like chickens. Parvalbumin Gal d 8 is typically found in the wing or thigh. Other allergens, like enolase (Gal d 9) and aldolase (Gal d 10), are isolated to the white meat.
- In crocodile meat. I must admit—I did not know that one could eat crocodile meat, but after some research I learned that in fact only the tail is eaten. Some people say its flavor resembles that of chicken, frogs, or fish. Perhaps this explains what I consider to be a rather exotic example of cross-reactivity.

The following story about a thirteen-year-old boy appeared in the journal *Pediatrics* in 2017 and ushered in a wealth of research attempting to identify the allergen responsible for his anaphylaxis. He was diagnosed with a chicken allergy at age five and a turkey allergy at age seven. Whenever he ate these foods, he immediately had an anaphylactic reaction. Ingesting dishes contaminated with chicken or turkey meat caused the same severe symptoms.

His father, the head chef in a restaurant, decided one day to make him something with crocodile meat. From the first bite, his son broke out in hives. His lips and throat began to swell and he started having trouble breathing. His parents quickly intervened and injected him with epinephrine. He was monitored for four hours. The doctors thought long and hard about this mysterious reaction and tried to hunt down what had caused it. A study published in 2018 by another research team proved that the culprit protein in our case was a parvalbumin found in the tail muscles of *Alligator mississippiensis*. Cross-reactivity in this instance is due to the structural similarities (94–100 percent) between crocodile and chicken parvalbumins.

In another observation that is no less astonishing, a nine-year-old child who was allergic to fish (apart from swordfish and tuna) also had an anaphylactic response to eating crocodile meat.

CHAPTER 8

Allergy Snapshots

Sometimes all it takes is a few minutes to deliver a short but specific piece of information. So here's a collection of little facts that hopefully will stick in your mind.

- Did you know that we shed between 70 and 140 mg of dead skin cells every day? Well! That small quantity is enough to feed several thousand dust mites for three months.
  - One gram of mattress dust contains around 2,000 dust mites.
  - The house dust mite ranges in size from 170 to 500 microns. 1 micron = 1 thousandth of a millimeter.
  - If you're wondering how fast a dust mite can move, the answer is 2 feet (60 cm) per hour. Dust mites also hitch rides on fabric fibers, particularly those in mattresses, thanks to suckers and hooks on the ends of their eight legs.

- Are you asking yourself where dust mite allergens are found? The answer is in their excrement. Oh, yes! They produce around twenty to forty small droppings per day and each one contains between 0.1 and 10 nanograms of the major dust mite allergen Der p 1. This allergen is destroyed by 140°F (60°C) C heat, which is why sheets should be washed at this temperature. Remember that in order to get rid of dust mite allergens completely, dust mites need to be killed and then vacuumed up or washed away along with their droppings.

- *Cheyletus eruditus* is a little plumper than its friend the domestic dust mite. It also doesn't play well with them. Instead, it crushes them with its powerful jaws and then eats them, leaving only the mites' shells behind. This predator has the potential to be a weapon of mass dust mite destruction and a hero of allergy prevention, except for one thing: it is suspected of being highly allergenic.

- Why should you worry about baby wipes? First of all, let's back up a little bit. Baby wipes in the United States sometimes contain methylisothiazolinone (MI), and there are many cases of contact eczema linked to this allergen. It is also found in many soaps and hair treatments. Unfortunately, these infamous wipes contain another allergen: phenoxyethanol. This preservative is highly controversial because of its effects on reproduction and should not be present in baby wipes. In many countries, such as France, the presence of phenoxyethanol must be included in a list of non-rinsed ingredients on every package of wipes. Some countries, such as France, warn that if phenoxyethanol is present, those wipes should not be used on children under three. Also keep in mind that depending on the brand, baby wipes may contain other allergenic substances like fragrances, lanolin, and acrylates (a filmogenic agent).

- Allergy to guar gum can cause severe reactions including anaphylaxis. This food additive is found in sauces, baked goods, and many gluten-free products.
- Pumpkin seeds are a good source of polyunsaturated fatty acids, but they may also trigger violent allergic reactions. Their allergens are resistant to heat and digestion, which is why they are capable of provoking anaphylaxis.
- Olives are an important part of Mediterranean food culture and are used in a variety of traditional dishes. The first observation of an olive allergy was in 2009. A twenty-eight-year-old man who knew he was allergic to dust mites and olive tree pollen was eating olives when he suddenly broke out in hives. His lips also started to swell. The verdict was clear from the positive skin tests—strangely, though, when this man ingested olive oil as part of a supervised oral food challenge, he did not experience any allergy symptoms.

- "How about some herbal tea?" "No thanks, I'm allergic." Does this dialogue sound odd to you? Well, just know that this kind of allergy has indeed been reported. One woman in her thirties felt itching and had difficulty breathing one hour after drinking chamomile tea. She also developed swelling and generalized hives, which indicates just how severe her allergic reaction was. Most of the people who react to chamomile are already sensitive to composite pollen (mugwort) and are victims of cross-reactivity. Chamomile exposure can happen in many different ways, whether it be through the use of phytotherapy, laxatives, eye care products, or certain ointments.

- Many French families like to end their meal with a little bit of salad. But did you know that the first rare cases of lettuce allergy were reported less than ten years ago? Lettuce belongs to the Asteraceae family, just like mugwort and ragweed.

- Terrarium lovers and fans of spiders, scorpions, and other similarly lovely creatures may think more carefully about what they feed their pets after reading this. These little beasts feed primarily on live crickets, but these can cause asthma and rhinitis in humans. The allergen is found in the cricket's body, as described in a 2014 article in the *Revue française d'allergologie*.

- You sneeze, but how fast? A group of curious scientists determined that the speed of a sneeze is 10 miles/hour

(16 km/hour) and it may go even faster depending on the person's weight.

- Here's a note for people who love hypoallergenic ceramic jewelry and people allergic to nickel who think they should buy it: unfortunately, it contains vanadium, and you may very well be allergic to this ingredient, too! This pale gray metal is used in metal alloys, the chemical industry, orthopedic prostheses, and ceramic jewelry.

- An early mention of an immediate IgE-dependent allergic reaction to pine nuts appears in an article published in 1958. Over the past twenty years, this allergy has been diagnosed more and more frequently, particularly in children. This makes pine nuts what is called an emerging allergen. Observed symptoms can range from hives to severe anaphylaxis after consuming pine nuts in their natural form or hidden in pesto sauces. A metallic or bitter taste in the mouth after eating pine nuts is not the result of an allergy but is an unpleasant possibility nonetheless. This can last anywhere from two days to two weeks. At present, there is no tangible explanation for this, but it appears certain species native to China like *Pinus armandii* and *Pinus massoniana* are to blame. In 2012, the Chinese authorities took measures to stop these species from being exported. In 2010, the French Agency for Food, Environmental and Occupational Health & Safety (ANSES) published a warning about distinguishing between edible and inedible pine nut varieties. If someone you know is experiencing this taste disturbance, they should contact a poison control center and keep a sample of the pine nuts for analysis.

- Do you remember the television show *Skippy the Bush Kangaroo*? If the answer is yes, you may find it somewhat jarring to hear that kangaroo meat is now a specialty product that is growing in popularity along with ostrich, bison, and buffalo meat. Alas, adverse reactions to kangaroo meat are entirely possible. A twenty-three-year-old man experienced this for himself after his lips swelled up the first time he tasted red-necked wallaby meat. But that didn't stop him! The second time he ate it, he developed severe anaphylactic symptoms within thirty minutes.

- In the summertime, mold allergies are sometimes mistaken for reactions to grass seed pollen. Mold allergy symptoms can be triggered by a minimum concentration of 100 *Alternaria* spores per cubic meter or 3,000 *Cladosporium* spores per cubic meter.

- Cypress trees release pollen all over southern coastlines of the United States beginning in January or February. It's a time of year that is hard to forget for anyone with allergies living in the region. Most of these people experience rhinitis, asthma symptoms, and conjunctivitis every year, and if that wasn't enough, they also have to be mindful of cypress pollen's cross-reactivity with peaches and citrus fruit.

- Here's an easy way to tell if a child's rhinitis symptoms are allergy-related: kids with chronic allergies often have an itchy nose and will usually rub it up and down with the palm of their hand. Over time this creates a wrinkle across the bridge of the nose. This is a sign that your little one is probably suffering from a respiratory allergy, not a cold.

- "Allergic shiners" in children are often mistaken for undereye circles from a lack of sleep, but they are actually a sign that a child is prone to allergies. This discoloration under the eyes is usually accompanied by two or three folds along the lower eyelids. These are known as Dennie-Morgan lines.

- Potty training a young child is no easy affair, but when allergies get involved, it becomes an absolute nightmare—and the famous potty chair turns into the family's worst enemy. Allow me to set the scene: a child's parents applaud her first pee pee or poo poo in the potty chair, and then proudly tell everyone they know about it . . . and their little one relieves herself generously and joyously before the amazed eyes of her audience. Then one day the mood is dampened when itchy red bumps of contact eczema suddenly cover her bottom. If the connection between the plastic of the potty chair and the dermatitis in question is not made quickly, this irritation can become chronic and last for several months.

What about adults?

Grown-ups' bottoms aren't safe from this allergy, either, but the culprits are not the same. In their case, contact eczema could be caused by a toilet seat made from pine (positive test for colophony), alder, or teak. Certain synthetic materials like polypropylene can also cause issues. Ingredients in polyurethane like isocyanates and diaminodiphenylmethane, a hardening agent, are known to trigger allergic reactions, too. The same is true for formaldehyde and isothiazolinone derivatives in cleaning products.

- A 2018 study found that the presence of a dog or cat during a baby's first year meant that the child was less likely to have allergies between the ages of seven and nine.
- The impact of global warming and pollution on pollen grains is far from negligible. Urban and industrial pollution modifies pollen's structure and composition, making it more "aggressive." The significant climate change observed in recent years has also influenced when plants bloom. Warmer winters in particular cause plants to bloom earlier and for longer periods of time. Pollen allergies in the United States affect around 19 percent of children and 26 percent of adults.
- Essential oils are extremely popular and seem to receive praise and media attention just about everywhere, but they're not as innocent as they appear. In reality, they are the invisible enemies of people with asthma and allergies. Here is a list of the most allergenic essential oils:

- Tea tree oil can cause severe contact eczema. Even if you do not notice any skin irritation when you apply it, it should not be used on skin in a concentration higher than 10 percent, if you have to use it at all.
- Contact eczema can also be triggered by eucalyptus essential oil, which is typically used in aromatherapy and some household products.
- Thirty percent of people with a fragrance allergy will also be sensitive to lavender essential oil, so it should be used with caution.
- Peppermint causes asthma symptoms and skin hypersensitivity.
- In 2015, Dr. Frédéric de Blay and his team studied the impact of spraying the air with a blend of one well-known brand's forty-one essential oils. They found that the concentration of limonene in the ambient air triggered asthma attacks in people prone to allergies. On top of that, as a result of oxidation, the mixture of essential oils also generated formaldehyde, a volatile organic compound (VOC) that is a major irritant and highly allergenic.
- I sneeze whenever I'm plucking my eyebrows. Is this an allergy?
  - Our bodies have twelve pairs of cranial nerves that originate in the brain stem. Some have sensory functions and others help our body make certain movements. The rest of them do a little of both. The

trigeminal nerve (fifth cranial nerve) is one of these. It allows us to bite, chew, and swallow, and also helps us feel pain or when something is touching our body. This nerve branches out over the face and one of these branches innervates the periorbital area. When we pluck our eyebrows, we are stimulating this portion of the trigeminal nerve. This is what triggers the sneezing reflex, not an allergy.

- My cousin told me she's allergic to the sun. She always sneezes when she looks at it. Is this really an allergy?
  - Believe it or not, this is an inherited reflex that is observed in around one-quarter of the general population. The medical term for it is photic sneeze reflex.* The most probable reason for this is signal interference between the optic nerve and its neighbor, the trigeminal nerve. When it is overstimulated by sunlight, the optic nerve causes the pupil to contract and the trigeminal nerve triggers a sneeze. This condition may seem laughable, but it can be disastrous for drivers and pilots. Accidents can happen so quickly when someone sneezes. . . .

- Ever heard of a grass juice allergy?
  - It was long thought that if someone developed rhinitis symptoms while mowing the lawn or handling fresh-cut grass, then that person was allergic to grass seed

---

* Or Autosomal Dominant Compelling Helio-Ophthalmic Outburst (ACHOO).

pollen. Recently, however, allergists have confirmed the existence of an allergy to grass juice that features its own set of respiratory reactions and have also worked to pinpoint which allergens are to blame.

- In 2019, an article appeared in the *Revue française d'allergologie* containing four clinical observations. The patients had either tested negative for airborne allergens or had tested positive for grass seed or birch tree pollen. All of the subjects, however, had positive prick tests for fresh-cut grass. The symptoms observed were generally rhinitis accompanied by asthma attacks and/or hives while mowing the lawn or handling fresh-cut grass in the spring and summer. The protein in the grass extract used for the prick test is present in the leaves of grassy plants and not in the pollen. It is a subunit of rubisco, a chloroplastic protein that makes up nearly 50 percent of the protein contained in the leaves.
- Now you'll know what to say if someone asks you about grass juice allergy! It has everything to do with leaf protein and nothing to do with pollen or mold.
- Playing the clarinet . . .
  - Who would have thought that playing a reed instrument could trigger contact allergies? And yet this is exactly what happened to a ten-year-old clarinet player. Whenever he played, he would develop eczema on his lower lip where it made contact with the cane reed. The boy had been diagnosed with atopic asthma

at age three. He was also allergic to grass seed pollen and in the process of following a desensitization protocol. Skin tests were performed with sawdust and an extract from the clarinet reed, which was made from *Arundo donax* cane. The boy's positive reaction persisted for several weeks! After getting rid of that cane reed, his initial symptoms disappeared except when he chewed on the tip of his wooden pencils or when his father was handling logs nearby. The cane in question is part of the grass family, which may explain this reaction in a child with a known allergy to the same kind of plant. Similar cases have been described involving the saxophone. The best solution for people with this problem is to use a polystyrene reed and avoid contact with objects like cane fishing rods and slats.

• Imagine: you're at a table with friends at a restaurant near the ocean. The sun is shining, the sky is azure blue. You're serenely sipping a margarita, or maybe a bottle of Mexican beer with a cute little slice of lime. As you squeeze the lime, a few drops of juice fall onto your arm. You quickly wipe them off. The next day you feel a burning sensation and notice red bubbles and a huge rash forming where you wiped the juice off with your hand. This is a form of phytophotodermatitis that some have called the "other" lime disease.* This skin reaction

---

* This has nothing to do with Lyme disease, a bacterial disease transferred by tick bites.

can take on impressive proportions, and the bubbles that form can resemble second- or third-degree burns.

- These symptoms are the result of a photochemical reaction between the skin, sunlight, and the furocoumarins contained in limes. The same thing can happen if you're lounging in the sun drinking a mojito that has already had lime juice added to it. Skin eruptions in this case can last several days or weeks and may leave pale or hyperpigmented scars.

- Phytophotodermatitis occurs when a photosensitizing plant substance comes into contact with the skin and is then exposed to UV sun rays. The skin feels like it's burning, rather than itching, and the rash only appears where contact with the plant substance was made.

- Other plants containing furocoumarins include parsnips, carrots, celery, mustard, parsley, and dill.

CHAPTER 9

Allergies, Science Fiction, and Comics

Does Darth Vader have asthma?

French pulmonologist Dr. Guillaume Colin—evidently a *Star Wars* fan—was so interested in the Sith Lord's respiratory troubles that he presented an unauthorized poster about his "research" on the subject at the French Language Pulmonology Congress in January 2018. I discovered his rather particular findings on Twitter.

The title of Dr. Colin's research project and the "real, fake" journal article he wrote is "Darth Vader: Asthmatic and He Doesn't Know It?" Members of this study's so-called "research team" are based in somewhat odd places including the Central Hospital of Coruscant, another facility in the Outer Rim, and one other at the South Pole of the Death Star. Like any seriously written journal article, in the introduction Dr. Colin describes his subject—Darth Vader, né Anakin Skywalker—and his problem, which he believes is none other than obstructive lung disease (asthma specifically). The researchers grounded their conclusions in a series of pulmonary function tests that Darth

Vader underwent on the Death Star before its destruction. "Spectral analysis" of his exhalations confirmed that their hertzian frequency matches wheezing observed in asthma patients. Dr. Colin offers several explanations for this phenomenon, including exposure to grass seed pollen and sulfur vapors.

> Humans in the Star Wars galaxy share the same biology and therefore the same diseases. Because of the Empire's censorship and thanks to the arrival of 5G on Earth, our pulmonologist colleagues on Coruscant turned to us for the publication of their new research. We previously published their 2018 study on the difficulty of using CPAP masks for Chewbaccas with sleep apnea.
>   In Anakin Skywalker's case, there are several arguments that point to asthma:
>   • PFT showing obstruction.
>   • Breath sounds reminiscent of wheezing.
>   • Exposure to allergens, dust, toxic vapors.
> The key question now is whether or not the Force and/or the Dark Side may have played a role in bronchodilation.

This is not the first time Dr. Colin has dared to shake things up. His first research poster* was entitled "A Comparative Study of CPAP Masks in Wookies." As he explains:

---

* Medical conferences bring health professionals together to share their latest research. In addition to attending presentations, conference participants can also consult summaries of recent journal articles on posters that are put on display.

"I got the idea from Banksy, an artist who used to sneak into museums and put up his own art next to famous paintings. I wondered if the same concept could be applied to medical conference posters. [. . .] Based on the way people reacted to my poster, I think that all of us who work in scientific research would benefit from a little more humor in our professional lives!"

Who knows? Perhaps one day you'll see a dermatologist or endocrinologist write an article on Chewbacca's hypertrichosis (excessive hair growth). Incidentally, this *Star Wars* character has already lent his name to a hairy beetle discovered in Papua New Guinea in 2016—*Trigonopterus chewbacca*.

Asthma, as we have discussed, is a respiratory disease linked to an inflammation of the bronchial mucus membrane. It is clinically characterized by three symptoms that occur together during an acute attack: shortness of breath, wheezing when exhaling, and coughing. Asthma diagnosis relies on a pulmonary function test (PFT) that shows evidence of obstruction and a reduced forced expiratory volume. This test also allows doctors to monitor the effectiveness of treatment, whether that be a daily corticosteroid spray or a combination of long-acting corticosteroids and bronchodilators. Treatment for an asthma attack requires the use of bronchodilators like salbutamol or terbutaline. In recent years, biotherapies like omalizumab have been used to stabilize severe asthma cases. Asthma education programs organized through hospitals or local organizations can help individuals with asthma learn how to manage their disease.

Farewell, Agrippine

Claire Bretécher left us at the age of seventy-nine in 2020. In 1972, she created *L'écho des savanes* with two other renowned cartoonists, Gotlib and Mandryka, and those comics (along with *Metal hurlant*) were by my side for all of the years I spent studying medicine. She was also the first person to receive the Grand Prix Spécial at the Angoulême International Comics Festival in 1983.

One of Bretécher's most famous comic book series follows the life of a teenage girl named Agrippine. When the seventh volume came out in 2004, the title caught my attention: *Allergies*. Now do you understand why I'm talking about her in this book?

Agrippine is often in crisis and frequently accompanied by Zonzon, her great-grandmother. I will freely admit that the comic strips in the book do not explicitly mention allergies, but in an interview in *Le Parisien* in October 2004, the cartoonist said she had been inspired by stories about allergies her girlfriends told her. Her timing couldn't have been better—she was focusing on diseases that were part of my everyday life as an allergist! In *Agrippine*, though, she uses the word "allergy" in the broader sense of the term, which many people do: I'm allergic to my teacher, to the color green, to humidity. . . . Wherever we use it, the expression always translates to a sort of immediate oversensitivity to or knee-jerk dislike of something. But is that really so far off from its use in a medical context? An allergy is, after all, an unnecessarily defensive reaction by the body to substances found in daily life. Either way, as Claire Bretécher puts it, "I'm sure there are plenty of people who will say that we shouldn't be laughing about allergies."

An article in *Le Monde* from January 2008 wondered why the cartoonist hadn't released any work since the release of *Allergies*. Bretécher responded that she was working on a new story, *Agrippine déconfite*, and that she was sweating blood and tears over it.

In her 2016 review of Claire Bretécher's work, Adeline Cuate observes that Agrippine only appears alone on the cover of two of the series' volumes: *Agrippine 1988* and *Allergies*. She also points out "Agrippine's obsession with her body; an obsession that extends even to her hair, as the reader discovers in the '*Tendance*' panel in volume 7. We also see this in the story about the slippers that are given to an old lady who doesn't like the color brown."

Let's look a little more closely at her comics, this time with a doctor's eye. The moment we open *Allergies*, Agrippine's grandma is giving her advice to win the battle against dust mites and we are immediately immersed in the world of allergies. The vocabulary the characters use makes it obvious that the cartoonist has spoken to an allergist. The stories continue, one after another, with everything from an allergic reaction to eating oysters in strawberry sauce to rhinitis caused by flowers. I have a slight preference for the piercing allergy in *"Bijoux de famille."* In another episode, Agrippine (who apparently has a peanut allergy) kisses her boyfriend, Persil Wagonnet, after he has eaten peanuts. Swelling ensues and her irresponsible companion runs away instead of helping her!

In *"Félina,"* our heroine dislikes a girl who comes over to her house. This girl is allergic to cats, so what better way to make her go away than to pull on a wool and cat hair sweater?

"Conflit social" details the adventures of Candida, the house-keeper, and her adventures with George Clooney, Agrippine's hedgehog. This animal gives Candida a runny nose and, as she says, "The hairs attach my antibodies to my mast cells and make the histamines come out!" It goes without saying that we should applaud the precision of her description of allergic rhinitis. Mast cells are indeed present in skin, lung, and digestive tissue. They play an essential role in immediate allergic reactions because when an IgE antibody on a mast cell binds to an allergen, this opens the immune cell's membrane and the cell releases a range of different substances including histamine.

At least according to my research, the theme of allergies has not been a source of great inspiration for cartoonists. I found a medical journal article about traumatic brain injuries in *Asterix and Obelix* and the portrayal of diseases in *The Adventures of Tintin*, but hardly anything about allergies, unless you count Captain Haddock's reaction to bee stings in "The Castafiore Emerald," an Italian comic book series called *Monster Allergy* about a young boy named Zick who is allergic to just about everything, and an article in *The Conversation* positing that Belgian cartoon character Gaston Lagaffe suffers from a hered-itary disease called Ehlers-Danlos syndrome that causes overly flexible joints and stretchy skin. Oddly enough, screenwriters seem more interested in allergies, and there are a number of films and television series—most of them crime shows—that include allergies in their storylines. If by chance this subject inspires you, illustrators of the world, let me assure you that in our specialty you will find plenty of material to work with—and we'd be happy to help!

Conclusion

Allergy medicine is such a rich specialty and I know it is definitely the one for me. This is fortunate, because we've been living side by side for over twenty-nine years! Honestly, I don't know if I chose it or if it chose me. What I love most about this job is solving allergy mysteries. In this book I decided to prioritize not only the allergies that affect daily life, but also the ones that are unexpected and, at times, downright astonishing. In my field, we always have to be thinking about the future, because what is totally new today will very likely become tomorrow's norm. When we look at the disease evolution, allergen identification, and diagnostic improvements that have taken place since the early twentieth century, we realize just how far we've already come. There is no doubt that years from now, other changes will come along, and the way allergists do things will be turned upside down once again, just as it has been in recent years.

The exponential increase in the number of people with allergies is no longer news. Even twenty years ago, it was estimated that one in four French people had an allergy. Today that number is one in three! This prevalence will grow, and projections estimate that in thirty years 50 percent of French people will be allergic to something. There are several factors that contribute to this phenomenon: an industrialized lifestyle, increasing pollution, and the consumption of fast food and processed food.

The detailed interview and carefully organized testing that are part of an allergist visit ensure an accurate diagnosis and save lives. I hope that reading about the diagnostic process has shown you how interesting it can be, and I hope that many more medical students will choose this fascinating profession that deals with so many different branches of medicine. My final wish for this book is that it would be a valuable source of helpful information for those of us who live with allergies every day.

APPENDICES

Appendix I

Recipes

Marie Lossy's story is far from ordinary. Two of her three children have multiple food allergies and were diagnosed at a very early age.

"My youngest is now twenty years old and a big guy who loves playing sports, but he has had severe, sometimes anaphylactic reactions to a large number of foods ever since he was a child: peanuts, celery, shellfish, wheat and other grains including gluten, all tree nuts, milk, eggs, lupine, mollusks, mustard, sesame, soy, sulfites, chestnuts, chickpeas, corn, flax, poppyseed, raw carrot and zucchini, as well as fruits (apricot, apple, pear, cherry) that cross-react with birch tree pollen. My oldest daughter is allergic to chia seeds, and if she eats raw or cooked pear she will have an asthma attack that can turn into anaphylaxis. Ingesting milk or dairy products (even traces) gives her vomiting, diarrhea, abdominal pain, dizziness, weakness, and intense fatigue. Her doctors think she may have FPIES."

When we inform parents that their child has a food allergy, they are often totally at a loss. They have to reorganize the way they live and eat. They have to inform friends and family and make sure they understand the severity of the risks involved and what foods need to be avoided. Far from letting herself be overwhelmed, this mom rolled up her sleeves and got to work! A fan of baking to begin with, she started making gluten-free breads that any professional would envy. For almost twenty years she has been inventing allergen-free recipes to delight her family, and shares them with the allergy community through her blog, *Allergique Gourmand*. She was kind enough to agree to select six of them to share in this book.

These recipes have no eggs, gluten, or milk and therefore do not contain any of the ingredients Marie's son is allergic to. Her daughter has grown up and left the nest like her other sister.

As far as other allergens go, you will need to go through each recipe to make sure you aren't allergic to anything in the list of ingredients. Now I'll hand things over to her.

Stuffed Tomatoes with Sunflower-Cucumber Cream

I'd like to invite you to prepare a delicious dish that requires no cooking and uses tomatoes, sunflower seeds, and cucumber. It does not contain gluten, milk, egg, or tree nuts.

One afternoon after soaking sunflower seeds, I decided I wanted to use them to make a little cream. I made my mixture without really knowing how it would turn out, but when I served it at the table and saw everyone taking seconds, I immediately thought this was something I should share.

To introduce it to you, I've chosen to use the cream as a tomato stuffing. Here's a fresh and exquisitely delicate recipe that I know you're going to love!

Preparation time: 15 minutes
Resting time: 2 hours in the refrigerator
Materials: Mixer and large bowl

2¾ ounces (75 g) sunflower seeds
4 fluid ounces (120 ml) hemp milk
3½ ounces (100 g) cucumber
Salt and pepper, to taste
Espelette pepper
Medium tomatoes
Chives

1. Soak the sunflower seeds for four hours in cold water. Drain and rinse, then add them to the mixer. Add the

hemp milk. Mix until the mixture is smooth. Pour this mixture into a large bowl.

2. Wash and finely dice the cucumber. Add to the sunflower seed mixture and combine. Season with salt, pepper, and Espelette pepper. Don't forget your chopped chives. Stir everything together.

3. Chill for two hours.

4. Next, core your tomatoes and fill them with your mixture. Garnish with a sprinkling of chives.

5. Enjoy.

Sweet Potato and Zucchini Fritters

We love sweet potatoes just as much in savory recipes as we do in sweet ones. I've made these gluten-, dairy-, and egg-free fritters with sweet potatoes, leeks, and mushrooms, and now I make them with zucchini, too.

I have added cumin to these fritters because it pairs so well with zucchini, and I've also included parsley from my garden. The end result is a plate of delicious fritters that are perfect alongside a generous salad or for eating on the go.

Cooking time: 15 minutes + 20 minutes
Preparation time: 15 minutes
Materials: Steamer, large bowl, and pan

    11¼ ounces (320 g) organic sweet potatoes
    6¾ ounces (190 g) organic zucchini
    Salt and pepper, to taste
    2 tablespoons organic quinoa flour
    ½ teaspoon organic cumin
    Organic parsley

1. Peel the sweet potatoes. Cut them into pieces and steam. Wash the zucchini and remove the ends.
2. Add the cooked sweet potato pieces to a large bowl and crush them with a fork.

3. Grate the raw zucchini. Add to the crushed sweet potatoes. Season with salt and pepper. Pour in the quinoa flour, cumin, and parsley. Stir together.

4. Lightly oil the pain. Place a metal cookie cutter in the pan and pour in a heaping tablespoon of the mixture. Smooth the top and cook for five minutes before flipping. Continue until you have used up all the batter.

5. Serve warm.

Chocolate Madeleines

When the weather is bad, I can't think of anything better than drinking a good cup of tea and munching on something sweet—like these gluten-, dairy-, and egg-free madeleines coated in a scrumptious little layer of chocolate!

The charm of a madeleine is in its little bump—the one we watch for while they're baking. Most people just cross their fingers and wait. I, on the other hand, attempt to avoid disappointment by leaving the kitchen, setting the timer, and not coming back until it rings.

But let's get back to that bump. I've done a little research and the keys to success are thermal shock and time to rest.

Preparation time: 15 minutes
Resting time: 1 night and 1 hour
Cooking time: 8 minutes at 425°F (220°C)

> 2 ounces (60 g) allergen-free margarine
> 4 fluid ounces (120 ml) hemp, buckwheat, or rice milk
> 2½ ounces (70 g) unrefined sugar
> 1½ ounces (40 g) tapioca starch
> 1½ ounces (40 g) buckwheat flour
> 1½ ounces (40 g) rice flour (half brown rice flour, half
>   white rice flour)
> 1 teaspoon (4 g) baking powder
> ¼ teaspoon baking soda

Ingredients continue on next page . . .

½ teaspoon vanilla powder (check label ingredients
   beforehand)
1 level teaspoon lemon zest
Allergen-free chocolate

1. In a large bowl, stir together the margarine and the hemp milk. Add the sugar and stir to blend.
2. In another bowl, combine the starch, flours, baking powder, and baking soda, then slowly pour this second mixture into the first large bowl, stirring to get rid of any lumps. Add the vanilla powder and the lemon zest . Stir until completely combined, then cover and refrigerate overnight.
3. The next day, grease your madeleine molds and fill them three-quarters of the way with yesterday's mixture and refrigerate for one hour.
4. Preheat the oven to 465°F (240°C)
5. Reduce the temperature to 430°F (220°C) and bake your madeleines on the bottom rack of the oven for eight minutes. Keep an eye on them—everyone's oven is different. And there you have it! The bump!
6. Take the madeleines out of the oven. Let cool. Melt the chocolate in a water bath. Dip the bottom of each madeleine in the chocolate and leave them on a baking tray to let the chocolate coating set. Then refrigerate.
7. Enjoy!

Original or Chocolate Langues de Chat Cookies

When I was little, every New Year's Eve at midnight my brothers and I would eat langues de chat cookies, with fruit juice for us and a flute of champagne for our parents. We used to love these dry little cookies. After a lot of research and testing, I arrived at this result . . . and I must say they're a true delight! They have all the crunchiness one expects from a langue de chat, and thanks to this recipe I can continue this family tradition without worrying about my child's allergies.

Preparation time: 15 minutes
Cooking time: 13 to 15 minutes at 355°F (180°C)
Materials: Baking tray, parchment paper, piping bag, mixer

    3 ounces (80 g) allergen-free margarine
    2¹⁄₁₀ ounces (60 g) organic unrefined sugar
    3 ounces (80 g) water
    3¹⁄₅ ounces (90 g) buckwheat flour
    1 tablespoon organic raw cocoa powder

1. Pour all of the ingredients into the mixer. Blend until smooth. Line the baking tray with parchment paper.
2. Transfer the mixture to a piping bag and pipe small rods onto the parchment paper. Make sure each one has plenty of room.

3. Bake for thirteen to fifteen minutes. The edges of the langues de chat should be a little brown. Remove the baking tray from the oven and cool. The cookies will continue to harden as they cool. Gently remove them from the parchment paper.

   Enjoy!

Organic Chocolate Coconut Spread

Dark chocolate, coconut, a little sugar, a little waiting, and you've got a delicious spread with no gluten, dairy, or egg to use on whatever you want!

This recipe will delight sweet lovers young and old. On a lovely slice of gluten-free bread, it is quite simply delicious. And the coconut flavor is not overpowering—just right.

For best results, I recommend making this spread in the morning to enjoy in the afternoon. The more it rests, the more time the flavors have to develop. Since the recipe contains margarine, it may take on a whitish color if you put it in the refrigerator, but this will not affect the taste: that's just the fat solidifying because of the cold.

Preparation time: 25 minutes
Resting time: 4 hours

　　5⅓ ounces (150 g) 75% cocoa chocolate
　　1 ounce (30 g) allergen-free margarine
　　1 tablespoon organic raw cocoa powder
　　3 ounces (80 g) organic coconut milk
　　4 tablespoons organic grated coconut
　　1½ ounces (40 g) organic unrefined sugar

1. Place the chocolate and margarine in a large bowl. Melt in a water bath. Stir together.

2. Turn off the heat. Remove the bowl from the water bath and add the cocoa powder, coconut milk, grated coconut, and sugar. Stir together until smooth.
3. Pour the spread into a jar with a sealing lid and store somewhere cool for four hours.
4. The longer the spread rests, the more prominent the flavors will be.
5. Enjoy on a thick slice of gluten-free toast.

Homemade Plant-Based Milk

For children over one and lactose-intolerant adults without allergies to tree nuts.

Materials: blender and large bowl

> 3½ ounces (100 g) almonds, hazelnuts, or a mixture of
>   the two
> 1 quart (1 l) water

1. Soak the almonds in water overnight. The next day, rinse them in clean water. Place in a blender with 1 quart (1 liter) of water. Blend until smooth. Pause the machine when necessary.
2. Filter the drink into a glass bottle. Store in the refrigerator for up to 3 days.*

Note

Below is the list of food allergens that must appear on food packaging labels in the United States.

1. Milk	6. Soy
2. Egg	7. Sesame
3. Peanut	8. Fish
4. Tree nut	9. Crustacean shellfish
5. Wheat	

---

* Talk to your doctor about calcium supplements.

Appendix II

Websites and mobile applications: Allergies 4.0

These days, you have to be plugged in. There is an abundance of information about allergies crawling all over the internet, but how do you find your way through it? Here is a selection of extremely useful websites and applications to help put you on the right path.

Allergy-related organizations and websites

Many people with allergies struggle with feeling alone when dealing with their illness. Here are several organizations that are always ready to help.

Allergy & Asthma Network
    https://allergyasthmanetwork.org/
Allergy Home
    www.allergyhome.org
The American Academy of Allergy, Asthma & Immunology (AAAAI)
    www.aaaai.org

American Academy of Pediatrics
    www.aap.org
*The American College of Allergy, Asthma & Immunology
    (ACAAI)*
    https://acaai.org/
American Partnership for Eosinophilic Disorders (APFED)
    www.apfed.org
Asthma and Allergy Foundation of America
    https://aafa.org/
American Academy of Dermatology
    www.aad.org
Immune Deficiency Foundation
    www.primaryimmune.org
Medical Alert Foundation
    www.medicalert.org
National Eczema Association for Science and Education
    www.nationaleczema.org
National Institute of Allergy and Infectious Diseases
    https://www.niaid.nih.gov/
World Allergy Organization
    https://www.worldallergy.org/

Food allergies

American Dietetic Association (ADA)
    www.eatright.org
Code Ana
    https://codeana.org/

FARE (Food Allergy Research & Education)
  https://www.foodallergy.org/
International FPIES Association (I-FPIES)
  www.fpies.org
Prevent Food Allergies
  https://www.preventallergies.org/

Allergy-friendly food websites

Many parents feel a little lost when we first tell them their child
has a food allergy. But there's no need to panic! You can find
plenty of websites offering everything from basic ingredients like
gluten-free flour to allergen-free baked goods, sauces, pasta, and
even prepackaged meals that are ready to eat. Your allergist can
help you choose depending on your allergies.

Feeding Your Kids Foundation
  https://feedingyourkids.org
Food & Friends
  https://foodandfriends.org
Kids with Food Allergies
  https://kidswithfoodallergies.org/
My Kids Lick the Bowl
  https://mykidslickthebowl.com

Pollen-related rhinitis

If you're looking for an app to track your allergy symptoms to see
if an allergy treatment is working, MASK-air (formerly known as
Pollen Diary) can do just that. This free application was created

by a team of allergists and allows you to record your symptoms for seven days and evaluates how your daily life improves (or not) with allergy treatment by having you answer a few questions. Available for download on your iPhone or Android.

Allergies and sleep apnea in children

Dr. Madiha Ellaffi, a passionate pulmonologist who specializes in allergies, happens to be the mother of four children who suffer from obstructive sleep apnea (OSA). To help families better understand this condition and reap the benefits of her expertise on the subject, she has created a free mobile app called *Woodchuck's Sleep* (available in the Google Play Store and the App Store).

Concise Bibliography

The studies and cases I reference in this book have been taken from a number of scientific journals. You can access further information about all of my sources by contacting Éditions du Rocher. *Note: If source has not been published in English, the original French source remains.*

- *Allergologia et Immunopathologia*
- *Allergologie en Pratique*
- *Allergology International*
- *Allergy*
- *Allergy, Asthma, and Clinical Immunology* (Official journal of the *Canadian Society of Allergy and Clinical Immunology*)
- *Annales de Dermatologie et de Vénéréologie*
- *Annals of Allergy, Asthma & Immunology*
- *BMJ*
- *Clinical and Molecular Allergy*
- *Contact Dermatitis*
- *European Annals of Allergy and Clinical Immunology*
- GERDA (skin allergy research group)

- *International Archives of Allergy and Immunology*
- *JAMA, The Journal of the American Medical Association*
- *Journal of Allergy and Clinical Immunology: In Practice*
- *Journal of Allergy and Clinical Immunology: In Practice Pediatrics*
- *Journal of Investigational Allergology and Clinical Immunology*
- *Journal of Sex & Marital Therapy*
- *Médecine et Droit*
- *New England Journal of Medicine*
- *OPA Pratique* (ENT specialists, pulmonologists, allergists)

Additional sources

Bretécher Claire, *Agrippine*, «Les allergies», Tome 7, Dargaud, 2004.

Caute, Adeline (McGill University & Dawson College), "Féminin, féminité et diversité dans les albums *Agrippine* de Claire Bretécher depuis 1995," Alternative francophone, vol.1, no 9, 2016, p. 5–18.

Cousins, Norman, *Anatomy of an Illness: As Perceived by the Patient*. New York: W.W. Norton, 1979.

Cousins, Norman, *Comment je me suis soigné par le rire*, Payot, coll. « Petite bibliothèque », 2003.

Goutey, Félix, "Un coléoptère porte le nom de Chewbacca," *Sciences et Avenir* (3 May 2019), https://www.sciencese tavenir.fr/animaux/arthropodes/un-coleoptere-porte-le -nom-de-chewbacca_103270

Quéquet, Catherine (Dr), *1001 allergies & intolérances*, Paris: Les éditions de l'opportun, 2017. https://oasis-allergie.org/2020/01/26/insolite-revelations-sur-lasthme-de-dark-vador/

Sampson H.A., Munoz-Furlong A., Campbell R.A., Franklin Adkinson Jr. N., Allan Bock S. et al., "Second symposium on the definition and management of anaphylaxis: Summary report-Second National Institute of Allergy and Infectious Disease/Food Allergy and Anaphylaxis Network symposium," *The Journal of Allergy and Clinical Immunology*, Feb. 2006; 117, p. 391–397.

Acronyms

A&A: Asthma and Allergies (French)

AFPRAL: French Association for the Prevention of Allergies

AFSCA: Belgian Federal Agency for the Safety of the Food Chain

ALPHO: Allergy to Neuromuscular Blocking Agents and Pholcodine Exposure

ANAFORCAL: French National Association for Continuing Education in Allergology

ANSES: French Agency for Food, Environmental and Occupational Health & Safety

ANSM: French National Agency for the Safety of Medicines and Health Products

CCDSHS: French National Data Committee in Humanities and Social Sciences

CEA: French College of Allergology Teachers

CFA: Francophone Congress of Allergology

CICBAA: Circle of Clinical and Biological Investigations in Food Allergy

CMPA: Cow's milk protein allergy

CNAF: French National Family Benefits Fund

CNGOF: French National College of Obstetricians and
   Gynecologists

CNOM: French Medical Council

DGAL: French Directorate General for Food

DGCCRF: French Directorate General for Competition
   Policy, Consumer Affairs, and Fraud Control

EFS: French National Blood Service

EGD: Esophagogastroduodenoscopy

ELFE: French Longitudinal Study of Children

EO: Essential oils

FA: Food allergies

FAO: Food and Agriculture Organization of the United
   Nations

FFAL: French Allergy Federation

FODMAPs: Fermentable oligo-, di-, monosaccharides, and polyols

FPIES: Food protein-induced enterocolitis syndrome

GST: Gold sodium thiosulfate

HA: Hypoallergenic

HACCP: Hazard Analysis Critical Control Point

HMP: Human Microbiome Project

IBD: Irritable bowel disease

IDT: Intradermal allergy tests

IgE: Immunoglobulin E

INED: French Institute for Demographic Studies

INN: International nonproprietary name

INSEE: French National Institute of Statistics and Economic
   Studies

INSERM: French National Institute of Health and Medical
 Research
InVS: French Institute for Public Health Surveillance
IVF: In vitro fertilization
LTP: Lipid transfer protein
MI: Methylisothiazolinone
NCGS: Non-celiac gluten sensitivity
NSAID: Non-steroidal anti-inflammatory drug
OFC: Oral food challenge
OIT: Oral immunotherapy
PEG: Polyethylene glycol
PFT: Pulmonary function tests
PGA: Poly(γ-glutamic acid)
PPD: Paraphenylenediamine
RAV: French Allergy Vigilance Network
RESIST: *Réseau d'entraide, soutien et informations sur la
 stérilisation tubaire* (support and information about
 permanent birth control)
RFA: *Revue française d'allergologie* (medical journal dedicated
 to allergies)
RNSA: France's National Network for Aerobiological
 Surveillance
ROAT: Repeated Open Application Test
SFA: French Allergy Society
SPLF: French Society of Respiratory Diseases
STD: Sexually transmitted diseases
SYFAL: French Syndicate of Allergists

THC: Delta-9-tetrahydrocannabinol
VOC: Volatile organic compound
WHO: World Health Organization

Acknowledgments

Nathalie Szapiro—you have been asking me to write a book like this for several years now. Here you go.

Christiane Capus, my wise reader, for always being so prompt and efficient no matter what I ask you to do.

A huge thank-you to Alex Dessinateur for his wonderful writing.

Laurence Coiffard, Madiha Ellaffi, and Sofia Dammak-Champeau for our first Instagram Live videos, and to Céline Couteau for our many discussions via LinkedIn.

Marie Lossy, an incomparable blogger and cook. I am so glad social media caused our professional paths to cross.

A big thank-you to Dr. Guillaume Colin for letting me in on the secret behind his Darth Vader research.

Thank you to Laura Zuili (Agence Caradine), Agnès Vidalie, and Éditions du Rocher, without whom this book would never have seen the light of day.

For the natto recipe: Thank you to Yves Legris (and to Vincent Héquet, I haven't forgotten the Hamamatsu photos).

Joseph . . . my reason . . .

Plume. My first green-eyed feline.

Notes

Please use this section to record any notes or to keep record of your allergic reactions.